BOB GREENE

THE BEST LIFE DIET

Daily Journal

REVISED AND UPDATED

SIMON & SCHUSTER

NEW YORK LONDON TORONTO SYDNEY

SIMON & SCHUSTER
Rockefeller Center
1230 Avenue of the Americas
New York, NY 10020

This Simon & Schuster hardcover edition January 2009

SIMON & SCHUSTER and colophon are registered trademarks
of Simon & Schuster, Inc.

For information about special discounts for bulk purchases,
please contact Simon & Schuster Special Sales at 1-800-456-6798
or business@simonandschuster.com.

Designed by Joel Avirom and Jason Snyder

Manufactured in the United States of America

10 9 8 7 6 5 4 3 2 1

ISBN-13: 978-1-4516-9748-3

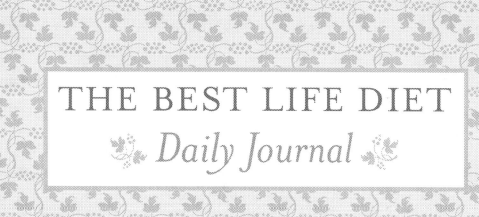

THE BEST LIFE DIET
Daily Journal

important to record any eating "episodes." These can be instances that are positive in nature, such as when you encounter a situation where you would typically overindulge and don't, or negative experiences, such as eating due to emotional turmoil. There is plenty of space dedicated for this journaling for each individual day. Don't forget to record the time of each episode and any pertinent information related to it. Logging this information can be enormously helpful for discovering patterns related to emotional eating and your behavior in general. Ultimately, this journal will help you to channel your energy toward healthy journaling, thus bringing you fulfillment as you explore ways to improve your life instead of overeating.

For additional support, be sure to read *The Best Life Diet* and log onto the supporting website at www.thebestlife.com.

General Health Information

(Consult with your physician before beginning this program.)

BEFORE

Weight _____   BLOOD PRESSURE: Systolic _____   Diastolic _____

Total Cholesterol _____   LDL _____   HDL _____   Blood Glucose _____

MEASUREMENTS (OPTIONAL):   Chest _____   Waist _____   Hips _____

NOTES _____

_____

_____

_____

_____

_____

_____

_____

_____

AFTER

Weight _____   BLOOD PRESSURE: Systolic _____   Diastolic _____

Total Cholesterol _____   LDL _____   HDL _____   Blood Glucose _____

MEASUREMENTS (OPTIONAL):   Chest _____   Waist _____   Hips _____

NOTES _____

_____

_____

_____

_____

_____

_____

_____

_____

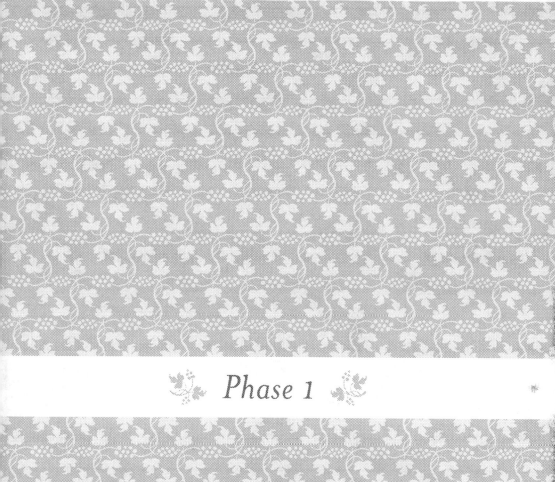

Phase 1

ACTIVITY LEVEL: 0   1   2   3   4   5

Aerobic minutes or steps/day _____

Did you meet your aerobic/step goal?   Y   N
NOTES _____

STRENGTH TRAINING

Exercise								
Weight								
Reps								
Sets								

Did you meet your strength-training goal?   Y   N
NOTES _____

Eating cutoff time: _____ : _____   Bedtime: _____ : _____

Did you cut off eating at least two hours before bedtime?   Y   N
NOTES _____

Did you eat three meals (including a nutritious breakfast) and at least one snack?   Y   N
NOTES _____

Did you eliminate the six problem foods from your diet?   Y   N
NOTES _____

Did you drink at least six 8-ounce glasses of water?   Y   N
NOTES _____

Did you take your vitamin supplements?   Y   N
NOTES _____

ACTIVITY LEVEL: 0   1   2   3   4   5

Aerobic minutes or steps/day _____

Did you meet your aerobic/step goal?   Y   N

NOTES _____

STRENGTH TRAINING

Exercise								
Weight								
Reps								
Sets								

Did you meet your strength-training goal?   Y   N

NOTES _____

Eating cutoff time: ____ ; ____   Bedtime: ____ ; ____

Did you cut off eating at least two hours before bedtime?   Y   N

NOTES _____

Did you eat three meals (including a nutritious breakfast) and at least one snack?   Y   N

NOTES _____

Did you eliminate the six problem foods from your diet?   Y   N

NOTES _____

Did you drink at least six 8-ounce glasses of water?   Y   N

NOTES _____

Did you take your vitamin supplements?   Y   N

NOTES _____

ACTIVITY LEVEL: 0   1   2   3   4   5

Aerobic minutes or steps/day _____

Did you meet your aerobic/step goal?   Y   N

NOTES _____

STRENGTH TRAINING

Exercise								
Weight								
Reps								
Sets								

Did you meet your strength-training goal?   Y   N

NOTES _____

Eating cutoff time: _____ ; _____   Bedtime: _____ : _____

Did you cut off eating at least two hours before bedtime?   Y   N

NOTES _____

Did you eat three meals (including a nutritious breakfast) and at least one snack?   Y   N

NOTES _____

Did you eliminate the six problem foods from your diet?   Y   N

NOTES _____

Did you drink at least six 8-ounce glasses of water?   Y   N

NOTES _____

Did you take your vitamin supplements?   Y   N

NOTES _____

ACTIVITY LEVEL: 0   1   2   3   4   5

Aerobic minutes or steps/day _____

Did you meet your aerobic/step goal?   Y   N

NOTES _____

STRENGTH TRAINING

Exercise								
Weight								
Reps								
Sets								

Did you meet your strength-training goal?   Y   N

NOTES _____

Eating cutoff time: _____:_____   Bedtime: _____:_____

Did you cut off eating at least two hours before bedtime?   Y   N

NOTES _____

Did you eat three meals (including a nutritious breakfast) and at least one snack?   Y   N

NOTES _____

Did you eliminate the six problem foods from your diet?   Y   N

NOTES _____

Did you drink at least six 8-ounce glasses of water?   Y   N

NOTES _____

Did you take your vitamin supplements?   Y   N

NOTES _____

ACTIVITY LEVEL: 0   1   2   3   4   5

Aerobic minutes or steps/day _____

Did you meet your aerobic/step goal?   Y   N
NOTES _____

STRENGTH TRAINING

Exercise								
Weight								
Reps								
Sets								

Did you meet your strength-training goal?   Y   N
NOTES _____

Eating cutoff time: _____:_____   Bedtime: _____:_____

Did you cut off eating at least two hours before bedtime?   Y   N
NOTES _____

Did you eat three meals (including a nutritious breakfast) and at least one snack?   Y   N
NOTES _____

Did you eliminate the six problem foods from your diet?   Y   N
NOTES _____

Did you drink at least six 8-ounce glasses of water?   Y   N
NOTES _____

Did you take your vitamin supplements?   Y   N
NOTES _____

ACTIVITY LEVEL: 0   1   2   3   4   5

Aerobic minutes or steps/day _____

Did you meet your aerobic/step goal?   Y N

NOTES _____

STRENGTH TRAINING

Exercise								
Weight								
Reps								
Sets								

Did you meet your strength-training goal?   Y N

NOTES _____

Eating cutoff time: _____:_____   Bedtime: _____:_____

Did you cut off eating at least two hours before bedtime?   Y N

NOTES _____

Did you eat three meals (including a nutritious breakfast) and at least one snack?   Y N

NOTES _____

Did you eliminate the six problem foods from your diet?   Y N

NOTES _____

Did you drink at least six 8-ounce glasses of water?   Y N

NOTES _____

Did you take your vitamin supplements?   Y N

NOTES _____

Weekly Summary

Total aerobic minutes/steps for the week _____

Did you meet your aerobic/step goal?   Y   N

Did you meet your strength-training goals for the week?   Y   N

How many days did you cut off your eating at least two hours before bedtime? _____

How many days did you eat three meals and at least one snack? _____

How many days did you eliminate the six problem foods? _____

How many days did you drink at least six 8-ounce glasses of water? _____

How many days did you take your vitamin supplements? _____

How was your week overall? _____

_____

_____

_____

_____

_____

_____

_____

_____

_____

_____

_____

_____

_____

_____

_____

_____

_____

_____

ACTIVITY LEVEL: 0   1   2   3   4   5

Aerobic minutes or steps/day _____

Did you meet your aerobic/step goal?   Y   N

NOTES _____

STRENGTH TRAINING

Exercise								
Weight								
Reps								
Sets								

Did you meet your strength-training goal?   Y   N

NOTES _____

Eating cutoff time: _____ : _____   Bedtime: _____ : _____

Did you cut off eating at least two hours before bedtime?   Y   N

NOTES _____

Did you eat three meals (including a nutritious breakfast) and at least one snack?   Y   N

NOTES _____

Did you eliminate the six problem foods from your diet?   Y   N

NOTES _____

Did you drink at least six 8-ounce glasses of water?   Y   N

NOTES _____

Did you take your vitamin supplements?   Y   N

NOTES _____

ACTIVITY LEVEL: 0   1   2   3   4   5

Aerobic minutes or steps/day _____

Did you meet your aerobic/step goal?   Y   N

NOTES _____

STRENGTH TRAINING

Exercise								
Weight								
Reps								
Sets								

Did you meet your strength-training goal?   Y   N

NOTES _____

Eating cutoff time: _____ : _____   Bedtime: _____ : _____

Did you cut off eating at least two hours before bedtime?   Y   N

NOTES _____

Did you eat three meals (including a nutritious breakfast) and at least one snack?   Y   N

NOTES _____

Did you eliminate the six problem foods from your diet?   Y   N

NOTES _____

Did you drink at least six 8-ounce glasses of water?   Y   N

NOTES _____

Did you take your vitamin supplements?   Y   N

NOTES _____

ACTIVITY LEVEL: 0   1   2   3   4   5

Aerobic minutes or steps/day _____

Did you meet your aerobic/step goal?   Y   N
NOTES _____

STRENGTH TRAINING

Exercise								
Weight								
Reps								
Sets								

Did you meet your strength-training goal?   Y   N
NOTES _____

Eating cutoff time: ____:____   Bedtime: ____:____

Did you cut off eating at least two hours before bedtime?   Y   N
NOTES _____

Did you eat three meals (including a nutritious breakfast) and at least one snack?   Y   N
NOTES _____

Did you eliminate the six problem foods from your diet?   Y   N
NOTES _____

Did you drink at least six 8-ounce glasses of water?   Y   N
NOTES _____

Did you take your vitamin supplements?   Y   N
NOTES _____

ACTIVITY LEVEL: 0   1   2   3   4   5

Aerobic minutes or steps/day _____

Did you meet your aerobic/step goal?   Y   N

NOTES _____

_____

STRENGTH TRAINING

Exercise								
Weight								
Reps								
Sets								

Did you meet your strength-training goal?   Y   N

NOTES _____

_____

Eating cutoff time: _____ : _____   Bedtime: _____ : _____

Did you cut off eating at least two hours before bedtime?   Y   N

NOTES _____

_____

Did you eat three meals (including a nutritious breakfast) and at least one snack?   Y   N

NOTES _____

_____

Did you eliminate the six problem foods from your diet?   Y   N

NOTES _____

_____

Did you drink at least six 8-ounce glasses of water?   Y   N

NOTES _____

_____

Did you take your vitamin supplements?   Y   N

NOTES _____

_____

ACTIVITY LEVEL: 0 1 2 3 4 5

Aerobic minutes or steps/day _____

Did you meet your aerobic/step goal?   Y N

NOTES _____

STRENGTH TRAINING

Exercise								
Weight								
Reps								
Sets								

Did you meet your strength-training goal?   Y N

NOTES _____

Eating cutoff time: ____:____   Bedtime: ____:____

Did you cut off eating at least two hours before bedtime?   Y N

NOTES _____

Did you eat three meals (including a nutritious breakfast) and at least one snack? Y N

NOTES _____

Did you eliminate the six problem foods from your diet?   Y N

NOTES _____

Did you drink at least six 8-ounce glasses of water?   Y N

NOTES _____

Did you take your vitamin supplements?   Y N

NOTES _____

ACTIVITY LEVEL: 0 1 2 3 4 5

Aerobic minutes or steps/day _____

Did you meet your aerobic/step goal? Y N

NOTES _____

STRENGTH TRAINING

Exercise								
Weight								
Reps								
Sets								

Did you meet your strength-training goal? Y N

NOTES _____

Eating cutoff time: ____:____   Bedtime: ____:____

Did you cut off eating at least two hours before bedtime? Y N

NOTES _____

Did you eat three meals (including a nutritious breakfast) and at least one snack? Y N

NOTES _____

Did you eliminate the six problem foods from your diet? Y N

NOTES _____

Did you drink at least six 8-ounce glasses of water? Y N

NOTES _____

Did you take your vitamin supplements? Y N

NOTES _____

ACTIVITY LEVEL: 0 1 2 3 4 5

Aerobic minutes or steps/day _____

Did you meet your aerobic/step goal?   Y N

NOTES _____

STRENGTH TRAINING

Exercise								
Weight								
Reps								
Sets								

Did you meet your strength-training goal?   Y N

NOTES _____

Eating cutoff time: ____ : ____   Bedtime: ____ : ____

Did you cut off eating at least two hours before bedtime?   Y N

NOTES _____

Did you eat three meals (including a nutritious breakfast) and at least one snack?   Y N

NOTES _____

Did you eliminate the six problem foods from your diet?   Y N

NOTES _____

Did you drink at least six 8-ounce glasses of water?   Y N

NOTES _____

Did you take your vitamin supplements?   Y N

NOTES _____

Weekly Summary

Total aerobic minutes/steps for the week   _____

Did you meet your aerobic/step goal?   Y   N

Did you meet your strength-training goals for the week?   Y   N

How many days did you cut off your eating at least two hours before bedtime?   _____

How many days did you eat three meals and at least one snack?   _____

How many days did you eliminate the six problem foods?   _____

How many days did you drink at least six 8-ounce glasses of water?   _____

How many days did you take your vitamin supplements?   _____

How was your week overall? _____

_____

_____

_____

_____

_____

_____

_____

_____

_____

_____

_____

_____

_____

_____

_____

_____

_____

ACTIVITY LEVEL: 0   1   2   3   4   5

Aerobic minutes or steps/day _____

Did you meet your aerobic/step goal?   Y   N

NOTES _____

STRENGTH TRAINING

Exercise								
Weight								
Reps								
Sets								

Did you meet your strength-training goal?   Y   N

NOTES _____

Eating cutoff time: ____:____   Bedtime: ____:____

Did you cut off eating at least two hours before bedtime?   Y   N

NOTES _____

Did you eat three meals (including a nutritious breakfast) and at least one snack?   Y   N

NOTES _____

Did you eliminate the six problem foods from your diet?   Y   N

NOTES _____

Did you drink at least six 8-ounce glasses of water?   Y   N

NOTES _____

Did you take your vitamin supplements?   Y   N

NOTES _____

ACTIVITY LEVEL: 0   1   2   3   4   5

Aerobic minutes or steps/day _____

Did you meet your aerobic/step goal?   Y   N

NOTES _____

_____

STRENGTH TRAINING

Exercise								
Weight								
Reps								
Sets								

Did you meet your strength-training goal?   Y   N

NOTES _____

_____

Eating cutoff time: _____ : _____   Bedtime: _____ : _____

Did you cut off eating at least two hours before bedtime?   Y   N

NOTES _____

_____

Did you eat three meals (including a nutritious breakfast) and at least one snack?   Y   N

NOTES _____

_____

Did you eliminate the six problem foods from your diet?   Y   N

NOTES _____

_____

Did you drink at least six 8-ounce glasses of water?   Y   N

NOTES _____

_____

Did you take your vitamin supplements?   Y   N

NOTES _____

_____

ACTIVITY LEVEL: 0   1   2   3   4   5

Aerobic minutes or steps/day _____

Did you meet your aerobic/step goal?   Y   N
NOTES _____

STRENGTH TRAINING

Exercise								
Weight								
Reps								
Sets								

Did you meet your strength-training goal?   Y   N
NOTES _____

Eating cutoff time: _____ : _____   Bedtime: _____ : _____

Did you cut off eating at least two hours before bedtime?   Y   N
NOTES _____

Did you eat three meals (including a nutritious breakfast) and at least one snack?   Y   N
NOTES _____

Did you eliminate the six problem foods from your diet?   Y   N
NOTES _____

Did you drink at least six 8-ounce glasses of water?   Y   N
NOTES _____

Did you take your vitamin supplements?   Y   N
NOTES _____

ACTIVITY LEVEL: 0   1   2   3   4   5

Aerobic minutes or steps/day _____

Did you meet your aerobic/step goal?   Y   N

NOTES _____

STRENGTH TRAINING

Exercise								
Weight								
Reps								
Sets								

Did you meet your strength-training goal?   Y   N

NOTES _____

Eating cutoff time: _____ : _____   Bedtime: _____ : _____

Did you cut off eating at least two hours before bedtime?   Y   N

NOTES _____

Did you eat three meals (including a nutritious breakfast) and at least one snack? Y   N

NOTES _____

Did you eliminate the six problem foods from your diet?   Y   N

NOTES _____

Did you drink at least six 8-ounce glasses of water?   Y   N

NOTES _____

Did you take your vitamin supplements?   Y   N

NOTES _____

WEEK: DATE: PHASE 1

ACTIVITY LEVEL: 0   1   2   3   4   5

Aerobic minutes or steps/day _____

Did you meet your aerobic/step goal?   Y   N
NOTES _____

STRENGTH TRAINING

Exercise								
Weight								
Reps								
Sets								

Did you meet your strength-training goal?   Y   N
NOTES _____

Eating cutoff time: _____ : _____   Bedtime: _____ : _____

Did you cut off eating at least two hours before bedtime?   Y   N
NOTES _____

Did you eat three meals (including a nutritious breakfast) and at least one snack?   Y   N
NOTES _____

Did you eliminate the six problem foods from your diet?   Y   N
NOTES _____

Did you drink at least six 8-ounce glasses of water?   Y   N
NOTES _____

Did you take your vitamin supplements?   Y   N
NOTES _____

ACTIVITY LEVEL: 0 1 2 3 4 5

Aerobic minutes or steps/day _____

Did you meet your aerobic/step goal?   Y N

NOTES _____

STRENGTH TRAINING

Exercise								
Weight								
Reps								
Sets								

Did you meet your strength-training goal?   Y N

NOTES _____

Eating cutoff time: ____:____   Bedtime: ____:____

Did you cut off eating at least two hours before bedtime?   Y N

NOTES _____

Did you eat three meals (including a nutritious breakfast) and at least one snack?   Y N

NOTES _____

Did you eliminate the six problem foods from your diet?   Y N

NOTES _____

Did you drink at least six 8-ounce glasses of water?   Y N

NOTES _____

Did you take your vitamin supplements?   Y N

NOTES _____

ACTIVITY LEVEL: 0   1   2   3   4   5

Aerobic minutes or steps/day _____

Did you meet your aerobic/step goal?   Y   N

NOTES _____

STRENGTH TRAINING

Exercise								
Weight								
Reps								
Sets								

Did you meet your strength-training goal?   Y   N

NOTES _____

Eating cutoff time: ____:____   Bedtime: ____:____

Did you cut off eating at least two hours before bedtime?   Y   N

NOTES _____

Did you eat three meals (including a nutritious breakfast) and at least one snack?   Y   N

NOTES _____

Did you eliminate the six problem foods from your diet?   Y   N

NOTES _____

Did you drink at least six 8-ounce glasses of water?   Y   N

NOTES _____

Did you take your vitamin supplements?   Y   N

NOTES _____

Weekly Summary

Total aerobic minutes/steps for the week   _____

Did you meet your aerobic/step goal?   Y N

Did you meet your strength-training goals for the week?   Y N

How many days did you cut off your eating at least two hours before bedtime?   _____

How many days did you eat three meals and at least one snack?   _____

How many days did you eliminate the six problem foods?   _____

How many days did you drink at least six 8-ounce glasses of water?   _____

How many days did you take your vitamin supplements?   _____

How was your week overall? _____

_____

_____

_____

_____

_____

_____

_____

_____

_____

_____

_____

_____

_____

_____

_____

_____

_____

_____

WEEK: **DATE:**   **PHASE 1**

ACTIVITY LEVEL: 0   1   2   3   4   5

Aerobic minutes or steps/day _____

Did you meet your aerobic/step goal?   Y   N

NOTES _____

STRENGTH TRAINING

Exercise								
Weight								
Reps								
Sets								

Did you meet your strength-training goal?   Y   N

NOTES _____

Eating cutoff time: ____ : ____   Bedtime: ____ : ____

Did you cut off eating at least two hours before bedtime?   Y   N

NOTES _____

Did you eat three meals (including a nutritious breakfast) and at least one snack?   Y   N

NOTES _____

Did you eliminate the six problem foods from your diet?   Y   N

NOTES _____

Did you drink at least six 8-ounce glasses of water?   Y   N

NOTES _____

Did you take your vitamin supplements?   Y   N

NOTES _____

ACTIVITY LEVEL: 0   1   2   3   4   5

Aerobic minutes or steps/day _____

Did you meet your aerobic/step goal?   Y   N

NOTES _____

STRENGTH TRAINING

Exercise								
Weight								
Reps								
Sets								

Did you meet your strength-training goal?   Y   N

NOTES _____

Eating cutoff time: _____ : _____   Bedtime: _____ : _____

Did you cut off eating at least two hours before bedtime?   Y   N

NOTES _____

Did you eat three meals (including a nutritious breakfast) and at least one snack?   Y   N

NOTES _____

Did you eliminate the six problem foods from your diet?   Y   N

NOTES _____

Did you drink at least six 8-ounce glasses of water?   Y   N

NOTES _____

Did you take your vitamin supplements?   Y   N

NOTES _____

ACTIVITY LEVEL: 0   1   2   3   4   5

Aerobic minutes or steps/day _____

Did you meet your aerobic/step goal?   Y   N
NOTES _____

STRENGTH TRAINING

Exercise								
Weight								
Reps								
Sets								

Did you meet your strength-training goal?   Y   N
NOTES _____

Eating cutoff time: _____:_____   Bedtime: _____:_____

Did you cut off eating at least two hours before bedtime?   Y   N
NOTES _____

Did you eat three meals (including a nutritious breakfast) and at least one snack?   Y   N
NOTES _____

Did you eliminate the six problem foods from your diet?   Y   N
NOTES _____

Did you drink at least six 8-ounce glasses of water?   Y   N
NOTES _____

Did you take your vitamin supplements?   Y   N
NOTES _____

ACTIVITY LEVEL: 0   1   2   3   4   5

Aerobic minutes or steps/day _____

Did you meet your aerobic/step goal?   Y   N

NOTES _____

STRENGTH TRAINING

Exercise								
Weight								
Reps								
Sets								

Did you meet your strength-training goal?   Y   N

NOTES _____

Eating cutoff time: ____ : ____   Bedtime: ____ : ____

Did you cut off eating at least two hours before bedtime?   Y   N

NOTES _____

Did you eat three meals (including a nutritious breakfast) and at least one snack?   Y   N

NOTES _____

Did you eliminate the six problem foods from your diet?   Y   N

NOTES _____

Did you drink at least six 8-ounce glasses of water?   Y   N

NOTES _____

Did you take your vitamin supplements?   Y   N

NOTES _____

ACTIVITY LEVEL: 0   1   2   3   4   5

Aerobic minutes or steps/day _____

Did you meet your aerobic/step goal?   Y   N
NOTES _____

STRENGTH TRAINING

Exercise								
Weight								
Reps								
Sets								

Did you meet your strength-training goal?   Y   N
NOTES _____

Eating cutoff time: ____ : ____   Bedtime: ____ : ____

Did you cut off eating at least two hours before bedtime?   Y   N
NOTES _____

Did you eat three meals (including a nutritious breakfast) and at least one snack?   Y   N
NOTES _____

Did you eliminate the six problem foods from your diet?   Y   N
NOTES _____

Did you drink at least six 8-ounce glasses of water?   Y   N
NOTES _____

Did you take your vitamin supplements?   Y   N
NOTES _____

ACTIVITY LEVEL: 0   1   2   3   4   5

Aerobic minutes or steps/day _____

Did you meet your aerobic/step goal?   Y   N

NOTES _____

STRENGTH TRAINING

Exercise								
Weight								
Reps								
Sets								

Did you meet your strength-training goal?   Y   N

NOTES _____

Eating cutoff time: _____:_____   Bedtime: _____:_____

Did you cut off eating at least two hours before bedtime?   Y   N

NOTES _____

Did you eat three meals (including a nutritious breakfast) and at least one snack?   Y   N

NOTES _____

Did you eliminate the six problem foods from your diet?   Y   N

NOTES _____

Did you drink at least six 8-ounce glasses of water?   Y   N

NOTES _____

Did you take your vitamin supplements?   Y   N

NOTES _____

ACTIVITY LEVEL: 0   1   2   3   4   5

Aerobic minutes or steps/day _____

Did you meet your aerobic/step goal?   Y   N

NOTES _____

STRENGTH TRAINING

Exercise								
Weight								
Reps								
Sets								

Did you meet your strength-training goal?   Y   N

NOTES _____

Eating cutoff time: ____ ; ____   Bedtime: ____ ; ____

Did you cut off eating at least two hours before bedtime?   Y   N

NOTES _____

Did you eat three meals (including a nutritious breakfast) and at least one snack? Y   N

NOTES _____

Did you eliminate the six problem foods from your diet?   Y   N

NOTES _____

Did you drink at least six 8-ounce glasses of water?   Y   N

NOTES _____

Did you take your vitamin supplements?   Y   N

NOTES _____

Weekly Summary

Total aerobic minutes/steps for the week   _____

Did you meet your aerobic/step goal?   Y   N

Did you meet your strength-training goals for the week?   Y   N

How many days did you cut off your eating at least two hours before bedtime?   _____

How many days did you eat three meals and at least one snack?   _____

How many days did you eliminate the six problem foods?   _____

How many days did you drink at least six 8-ounce glasses of water?   _____

How many days did you take your vitamin supplements?   _____

How was your week overall? _____

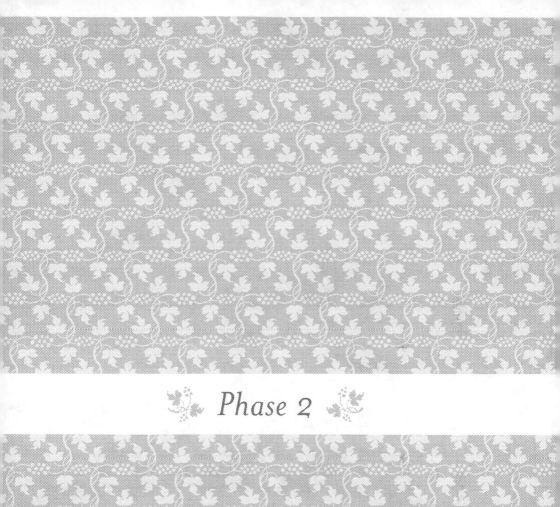

Phase 2

WEEK: DATE: PHASE 2

ACTIVITY LEVEL:　0　1　2　3　4　5

Aerobic minutes or steps/day _____

Did you meet your aerobic/step goal?　　　　　　　　　　　　　　Y　N
NOTES _____

STRENGTH TRAINING

Exercise								
Weight								
Reps								
Sets								

Did you meet your strength-training goal?　　　　　　　　　　　　Y　N
NOTES _____

Eating cutoff time: _____ : _____　　　Bedtime: _____ : _____

Did you cut off eating at least two hours before bedtime?　　　　　　Y　N

Did you eat three meals (including a nutritious breakfast) and at least one snack?　　Y　N

Did you eliminate the six problem foods from your diet?　　　　　　Y　N

Did you drink at least six 8-ounce glasses of water?　　　　　　　Y　N

Did you take your vitamin supplements?　　　　　　　　　　　　Y　N

　　　　　　　　　TIME
Breakfast　　　_____ : _____　Hunger rating before eating _____　Hunger rating after eating _____

Lunch　　　　_____ : _____　Hunger rating before eating _____　Hunger rating after eating _____

Dinner　　　　_____ : _____　Hunger rating before eating _____　Hunger rating after eating _____

Snack　　　　_____ : _____　Hunger rating before eating _____　Hunger rating after eating _____

Other meal/snack _____ : _____　Hunger rating before eating _____　Hunger rating after eating _____

Other meal/snack _____ : _____　Hunger rating before eating _____　Hunger rating after eating _____

Did you meet your hunger scale goals?　　　　　　　　　　　　Y　N
NOTES _____
_____

Write down the number of servings you had in each food group. For Anything Goes, just write down the total number of treat calories you had. For a refresher on what counts as a serving, see page 119 in *The Best Life Diet*. And to find out how many servings of grains, fruit, and the other food groups you should have daily (and how many Anything Goes Calories you get), look at the chart on page 119 of the book. (Remember, you can also track your intake and get feedback by joining www.thebestlife.com.)

	Breakfast	Lunch	Dinner	Snack	Other	Other
Grain/Starchy Vegetables						
Fruit						
Vegetables						
Dairy (preferably nonfat or 1%)						
Protein-Rich Foods						
Fat (preferably healthy)						
Anything Goes Calories						

Are your portions becoming more reasonable?   Y   N

NOTES_____

_____

Did you stay within your Anything Goes Calories for treats?   Y   N

NOTES_____

_____

_____

_____

_____

_____

_____

_____

_____

_____

_____

_____

_____

_____

_____

_____

_____

_____

ACTIVITY LEVEL: 0 1 2 3 4 5

Aerobic minutes or steps/day _____

Did you meet your aerobic/step goal? Y N

NOTES _____

_____

STRENGTH TRAINING

Exercise								
Weight								
Reps								
Sets								

Did you meet your strength-training goal? Y N

NOTES _____

_____

Eating cutoff time: ____ : ____   Bedtime: ____ : ____

Did you cut off eating at least two hours before bedtime? Y N

Did you eat three meals (including a nutritious breakfast) and at least one snack? Y N

Did you eliminate the six problem foods from your diet? Y N

Did you drink at least six 8-ounce glasses of water? Y N

Did you take your vitamin supplements? Y N

                    TIME

Breakfast   ____ : ____   Hunger rating before eating ____ Hunger rating after eating ____

Lunch   ____ : ____   Hunger rating before eating ____ Hunger rating after eating ____

Dinner   ____ : ____   Hunger rating before eating ____ Hunger rating after eating ____

Snack   ____ : ____   Hunger rating before eating ____ Hunger rating after eating ____

Other meal/snack ____ : ____   Hunger rating before eating ____ Hunger rating after eating ____

Other meal/snack ____ : ____   Hunger rating before eating ____ Hunger rating after eating ____

Did you meet your hunger scale goals? Y N

NOTES _____

_____

Write down the number of servings you had in each food group. For Anything Goes, just write down the total number of treat calories you had. For a refresher on what counts as a serving, see page 119 in *The Best Life Diet*. And to find out how many servings of grains, fruit, and the other food groups you should have daily (and how many Anything Goes Calories you get), look at the chart on page 119 of the book. (Remember, you can also track your intake and get feedback by joining www.thebestlife.com.)

	Breakfast	Lunch	Dinner	Snack	Other	Other
Grain/Starchy Vegetables						
Fruit						
Vegetables						
Dairy (preferably nonfat or 1%)						
Protein-Rich Foods						
Fat (preferably healthy)						
Anything Goes Calories						

Are your portions becoming more reasonable?   Y   N

NOTES _____

_____

Did you stay within your Anything Goes Calories for treats?   Y   N

NOTES _____

_____

_____

_____

_____

_____

_____

_____

_____

_____

_____

_____

_____

_____

_____

_____

_____

_____

ACTIVITY LEVEL: 0   1   2   3   4   5

Aerobic minutes or steps/day _____

Did you meet your aerobic/step goal?   Y   N

NOTES _____

STRENGTH TRAINING

Exercise								
Weight								
Reps								
Sets								

Did you meet your strength-training goal?   Y   N

NOTES _____

Eating cutoff time: ____ : ____   Bedtime: ____ : ____

Did you cut off eating at least two hours before bedtime?   Y   N

Did you eat three meals (including a nutritious breakfast) and at least one snack?   Y   N

Did you eliminate the six problem foods from your diet?   Y   N

Did you drink at least six 8-ounce glasses of water?   Y   N

Did you take your vitamin supplements?   Y   N

                   TIME

Breakfast   ____ : ____   Hunger rating before eating ____ Hunger rating after eating ____

Lunch   ____ : ____   Hunger rating before eating ____ Hunger rating after eating ____

Dinner   ____ : ____   Hunger rating before eating ____ Hunger rating after eating ____

Snack   ____ : ____   Hunger rating before eating ____ Hunger rating after eating ____

Other meal/snack ____ : ____   Hunger rating before eating ____ Hunger rating after eating ____

Other meal/snack ____ : ____   Hunger rating before eating ____ Hunger rating after eating ____

Did you meet your hunger scale goals?   Y   N

NOTES _____

_____

Write down the number of servings you had in each food group. For Anything Goes, just write down the total number of treat calories you had. For a refresher on what counts as a serving, see page 119 in *The Best Life Diet*. And to find out how many servings of grains, fruit, and the other food groups you should have daily (and how many Anything Goes Calories you get), look at the chart on page 119 of the book. (Remember, you can also track your intake and get feedback by joining www.thebestlife.com.)

	Breakfast	Lunch	Dinner	Snack	Other	Other
Grain/Starchy Vegetables						
Fruit						
Vegetables						
Dairy (preferably nonfat or 1%)						
Protein-Rich Foods						
Fat (preferably healthy)						
Anything Goes Calories						

Are your portions becoming more reasonable?　　Y　N

NOTES _____

_____

Did you stay within your Anything Goes Calories for treats?　　Y　N

NOTES _____

_____

_____

_____

_____

_____

_____

_____

_____

_____

_____

_____

_____

_____

_____

_____

_____

ACTIVITY LEVEL: 0   1   2   3   4   5

Aerobic minutes or steps/day _____

Did you meet your aerobic/step goal?   Y   N

NOTES _____

_____

STRENGTH TRAINING

Exercise								
Weight								
Reps								
Sets								

Did you meet your strength-training goal?   Y   N

NOTES _____

_____

Eating cutoff time: ____:____   Bedtime: ____:____

Did you cut off eating at least two hours before bedtime?   Y   N

Did you eat three meals (including a nutritious breakfast) and at least one snack?   Y   N

Did you eliminate the six problem foods from your diet?   Y   N

Did you drink at least six 8-ounce glasses of water?   Y   N

Did you take your vitamin supplements?   Y   N

	TIME		
Breakfast	____:____	Hunger rating before eating ____	Hunger rating after eating ____
Lunch	____:____	Hunger rating before eating ____	Hunger rating after eating ____
Dinner	____:____	Hunger rating before eating ____	Hunger rating after eating ____
Snack	____:____	Hunger rating before eating ____	Hunger rating after eating ____
Other meal/snack	____:____	Hunger rating before eating ____	Hunger rating after eating ____
Other meal/snack	____:____	Hunger rating before eating ____	Hunger rating after eating ____

Did you meet your hunger scale goals?   Y   N

NOTES _____

_____

Write down the number of servings you had in each food group. For Anything Goes, just write down the total number of treat calories you had. For a refresher on what counts as a serving, see page 119 in *The Best Life Diet*. And to find out how many servings of grains, fruit, and the other food groups you should have daily (and how many Anything Goes Calories you get), look at the chart on page 119 of the book. (Remember, you can also track your intake and get feedback by joining www.thebestlife.com.)

	Breakfast	Lunch	Dinner	Snack	Other	Other
Grain/Starchy Vegetables						
Fruit						
Vegetables						
Dairy (preferably nonfat or 1%)						
Protein-Rich Foods						
Fat (preferably healthy)						
Anything Goes Calories						

Are your portions becoming more reasonable?   Y   N

NOTES _____

_____

Did you stay within your Anything Goes Calories for treats?   Y   N

NOTES _____

_____

_____

_____

_____

_____

_____

_____

_____

_____

_____

_____

_____

_____

_____

_____

_____

ACTIVITY LEVEL: 0 1 2 3 4 5

Aerobic minutes or steps/day _____

Did you meet your aerobic/step goal?   Y N

NOTES _____

STRENGTH TRAINING

Exercise								
Weight								
Reps								
Sets								

Did you meet your strength-training goal?   Y N

NOTES _____

Eating cutoff time: ____ : ____   Bedtime: ____ : ____

Did you cut off eating at least two hours before bedtime?   Y N

Did you eat three meals (including a nutritious breakfast) and at least one snack?   Y N

Did you eliminate the six problem foods from your diet?   Y N

Did you drink at least six 8-ounce glasses of water?   Y N

Did you take your vitamin supplements?   Y N

                    TIME

Breakfast   ____ : ____   Hunger rating before eating ____   Hunger rating after eating ____

Lunch   ____ : ____   Hunger rating before eating ____   Hunger rating after eating ____

Dinner   ____ : ____   Hunger rating before eating ____   Hunger rating after eating ____

Snack   ____ : ____   Hunger rating before eating ____   Hunger rating after eating ____

Other meal/snack ____ : ____   Hunger rating before eating ____   Hunger rating after eating ____

Other meal/snack ____ : ____   Hunger rating before eating ____   Hunger rating after eating ____

Did you meet your hunger scale goals?   Y N

NOTES _____

Write down the number of servings you had in each food group. For Anything Goes, just write down the total number of treat calories you had. For a refresher on what counts as a serving, see page 119 in *The Best Life Diet*. And to find out how many servings of grains, fruit, and the other food groups you should have daily (and how many Anything Goes Calories you get), look at the chart on page 119 of the book. (Remember, you can also track your intake and get feedback by joining www.thebestlife.com.)

	Breakfast	Lunch	Dinner	Snack	Other	Other
Grain/Starchy Vegetables						
Fruit						
Vegetables						
Dairy (preferably nonfat or 1%)						
Protein-Rich Foods						
Fat (preferably healthy)						
Anything Goes Calories						

Are your portions becoming more reasonable?   Y   N

NOTES _____

_____

Did you stay within your Anything Goes Calories for treats?   Y   N

NOTES _____

_____

_____

_____

_____

_____

_____

_____

_____

_____

_____

_____

_____

_____

_____

_____

_____

_____

_____

ACTIVITY LEVEL: 0   1   2   3   4   5

Aerobic minutes or steps/day _____

Did you meet your aerobic/step goal?   Y   N

NOTES _____

STRENGTH TRAINING

Exercise								
Weight								
Reps								
Sets								

Did you meet your strength-training goal?   Y   N

NOTES _____

Eating cutoff time: ____ : ____   Bedtime: ____ : ____

Did you cut off eating at least two hours before bedtime?   Y   N

Did you eat three meals (including a nutritious breakfast) and at least one snack?   Y   N

Did you eliminate the six problem foods from your diet?   Y   N

Did you drink at least six 8-ounce glasses of water?   Y   N

Did you take your vitamin supplements?   Y   N

                   TIME

Breakfast   ____ : ____   Hunger rating before eating ____   Hunger rating after eating ____

Lunch   ____ : ____   Hunger rating before eating ____   Hunger rating after eating ____

Dinner   ____ : ____   Hunger rating before eating ____   Hunger rating after eating ____

Snack   ____ : ____   Hunger rating before eating ____   Hunger rating after eating ____

Other meal/snack ____ : ____   Hunger rating before eating ____   Hunger rating after eating ____

Other meal/snack ____ : ____   Hunger rating before eating ____   Hunger rating after eating ____

Did you meet your hunger scale goals?   Y   N

NOTES _____

Write down the number of servings you had in each food group. For Anything Goes, just write down the total number of treat calories you had. For a refresher on what counts as a serving, see page 119 in *The Best Life Diet*. And to find out how many servings of grains, fruit, and the other food groups you should have daily (and how many Anything Goes Calories you get), look at the chart on page 119 of the book. (Remember, you can also track your intake and get feedback by joining www.thebestlife.com.)

	Breakfast	Lunch	Dinner	Snack	Other	Other
Grain/Starchy Vegetables						
Fruit						
Vegetables						
Dairy (preferably nonfat or 1%)						
Protein-Rich Foods						
Fat (preferably healthy)						
Anything Goes Calories						

Are your portions becoming more reasonable?   Y   N

NOTES _____

_____

Did you stay within your Anything Goes Calories for treats?   Y   N

NOTES _____

_____

_____

_____

_____

_____

_____

_____

_____

_____

_____

_____

_____

_____

_____

_____

_____

_____

WEEK: DATE: PHASE 2

ACTIVITY LEVEL: 0   1   2   3   4   5

Aerobic minutes or steps/day _____

Did you meet your aerobic/step goal?   Y   N

NOTES _____

STRENGTH TRAINING

Exercise								
Weight								
Reps								
Sets								

Did you meet your strength-training goal?   Y   N

NOTES _____

Eating cutoff time: ____ : ____   Bedtime: ____ : ____

Did you cut off eating at least two hours before bedtime?   Y   N

Did you eat three meals (including a nutritious breakfast) and at least one snack?   Y   N

Did you eliminate the six problem foods from your diet?   Y   N

Did you drink at least six 8-ounce glasses of water?   Y   N

Did you take your vitamin supplements?   Y   N

                         TIME

Breakfast   ____ : ____   Hunger rating before eating ____   Hunger rating after eating ____

Lunch   ____ : ____   Hunger rating before eating ____   Hunger rating after eating ____

Dinner   ____ : ____   Hunger rating before eating ____   Hunger rating after eating ____

Snack   ____ : ____   Hunger rating before eating ____   Hunger rating after eating ____

Other meal/snack ____ : ____   Hunger rating before eating ____   Hunger rating after eating ____

Other meal/snack ____ : ____   Hunger rating before eating ____   Hunger rating after eating ____

Did you meet your hunger scale goals?   Y   N

NOTES _____

_____

Write down the number of servings you had in each food group. For Anything Goes, just write down the total number of treat calories you had. For a refresher on what counts as a serving, see page 119 in *The Best Life Diet*. And to find out how many servings of grains, fruit, and the other food groups you should have daily (and how many Anything Goes Calories you get), look at the chart on page 119 of the book. (Remember, you can also track your intake and get feedback by joining www.thebestlife.com.)

	Breakfast	Lunch	Dinner	Snack	Other	Other
Grain/Starchy Vegetables						
Fruit						
Vegetables						
Dairy (preferably nonfat or 1%)						
Protein-Rich Foods						
Fat (preferably healthy)						
Anything Goes Calories						

Are your portions becoming more reasonable?   Y   N

NOTES_____

_____

Did you stay within your Anything Goes Calories for treats?   Y   N

NOTES_____

_____

_____

_____

_____

_____

_____

_____

_____

_____

_____

_____

_____

_____

_____

_____

_____

_____

Weekly Summary

Your weight: _____

Total aerobic minutes/steps for the week _____

Did you meet your aerobic/step goal?   Y   N

Did you meet your strength-training goals for the week?   Y   N

How many days did you cut off your eating at least two hours before bedtime? _____

How many days did you eat three meals and at least one snack? _____

How many days did eliminate the six problem foods? _____

How many days did you drink at least six 8-ounce glasses of water? _____

How many days did you take your vitamin supplements? _____

How many days did you meet your hunger scale goals? _____

How many days did you eat reasonable portions? _____

How many days did you stay within your Anything Goes Calories for treats? _____

How was your week overall? _____

_____

_____

_____

_____

_____

_____

_____

_____

_____

_____

_____

_____

ACTIVITY LEVEL: 0   1   2   3   4   5

Aerobic minutes or steps/day _____

Did you meet your aerobic/step goal?   Y   N

NOTES _____

_____

STRENGTH TRAINING

Exercise								
Weight								
Reps								
Sets								

Did you meet your strength-training goal?   Y   N

NOTES _____

_____

Eating cutoff time: _____ : _____   Bedtime: _____ : _____

Did you cut off eating at least two hours before bedtime?   Y   N

Did you eat three meals (including a nutritious breakfast) and at least one snack?   Y   N

Did you eliminate the six problem foods from your diet?   Y   N

Did you drink at least six 8-ounce glasses of water?   Y   N

Did you take your vitamin supplements?   Y   N

	TIME		
Breakfast	_____ : _____	Hunger rating before eating _____	Hunger rating after eating _____
Lunch	_____ : _____	Hunger rating before eating _____	Hunger rating after eating _____
Dinner	_____ : _____	Hunger rating before eating _____	Hunger rating after eating _____
Snack	_____ : _____	Hunger rating before eating _____	Hunger rating after eating _____
Other meal/snack	_____ : _____	Hunger rating before eating _____	Hunger rating after eating _____
Other meal/snack	_____ : _____	Hunger rating before eating _____	Hunger rating after eating _____

Did you meet your hunger scale goals?   Y   N

NOTES _____

_____

Write down the number of servings you had in each food group. For Anything Goes, just write down the total number of treat calories you had. For a refresher on what counts as a serving, see page 119 in *The Best Life Diet*. And to find out how many servings of grains, fruit, and the other food groups you should have daily (and how many Anything Goes Calories you get), look at the chart on page 119 of the book. (Remember, you can also track your intake and get feedback by joining www.thebestlife.com.)

	Breakfast	Lunch	Dinner	Snack	Other	Other
Grain/Starchy Vegetables						
Fruit						
Vegetables						
Dairy (preferably nonfat or 1%)						
Protein-Rich Foods						
Fat (preferably healthy)						
Anything Goes Calories						

Are your portions becoming more reasonable?   Y   N

NOTES _____

_____

Did you stay within your Anything Goes Calories for treats?   Y   N

NOTES _____

_____

_____

_____

_____

_____

_____

_____

_____

_____

_____

_____

_____

_____

_____

_____

_____

_____

_____

_____

ACTIVITY LEVEL: 0   1   2   3   4   5

Aerobic minutes or steps/day _____

Did you meet your aerobic/step goal?   Y   N

NOTES _____

STRENGTH TRAINING

Exercise								
Weight								
Reps								
Sets								

Did you meet your strength-training goal?   Y   N

NOTES _____

Eating cutoff time: _____:_____   Bedtime: _____:_____

Did you cut off eating at least two hours before bedtime?   Y   N

Did you eat three meals (including a nutritious breakfast) and at least one snack?   Y   N

Did you eliminate the six problem foods from your diet?   Y   N

Did you drink at least six 8-ounce glasses of water?   Y   N

Did you take your vitamin supplements?   Y   N

TIME

Breakfast   _____:_____   Hunger rating before eating _____ Hunger rating after eating _____

Lunch   _____:_____   Hunger rating before eating _____ Hunger rating after eating _____

Dinner   _____:_____   Hunger rating before eating _____ Hunger rating after eating _____

Snack   _____:_____   Hunger rating before eating _____ Hunger rating after eating _____

Other meal/snack _____:_____   Hunger rating before eating _____ Hunger rating after eating _____

Other meal/snack _____:_____   Hunger rating before eating _____ Hunger rating after eating _____

Did you meet your hunger scale goals?   Y   N

NOTES _____

_____

Write down the number of servings you had in each food group. For Anything Goes, just write down the total number of treat calories you had. For a refresher on what counts as a serving, see page 119 in *The Best Life Diet*. And to find out how many servings of grains, fruit, and the other food groups you should have daily (and how many Anything Goes Calories you get), look at the chart on page 119 of the book. (Remember, you can also track your intake and get feedback by joining www.thebestlife.com.)

	Breakfast	Lunch	Dinner	Snack	Other	Other
Grain/Starchy Vegetables						
Fruit						
Vegetables						
Dairy (preferably nonfat or 1%)						
Protein-Rich Foods						
Fat (preferably healthy)						
Anything Goes Calories						

Are your portions becoming more reasonable? Y N

NOTES _____

_____

Did you stay within your Anything Goes Calories for treats? Y N

NOTES _____

_____

_____

_____

_____

_____

_____

_____

_____

_____

_____

_____

_____

_____

_____

_____

_____

WEEK: **DATE:**   **PHASE 2**

ACTIVITY LEVEL: 0   1   2   3   4   5

Aerobic minutes or steps/day _____

Did you meet your aerobic/step goal?   Y   N

NOTES _____

_____

STRENGTH TRAINING

Exercise								
Weight								
Reps								
Sets								

Did you meet your strength-training goal?   Y   N

NOTES _____

_____

Eating cutoff time: ____ : ____   Bedtime: ____ : ____

Did you cut off eating at least two hours before bedtime?   Y   N

Did you eat three meals (including a nutritious breakfast) and at least one snack?   Y   N

Did you eliminate the six problem foods from your diet?   Y   N

Did you drink at least six 8-ounce glasses of water?   Y   N

Did you take your vitamin supplements?   Y   N

                              TIME

Breakfast   ____ : ____   Hunger rating before eating ____   Hunger rating after eating ____

Lunch   ____ : ____   Hunger rating before eating ____   Hunger rating after eating ____

Dinner   ____ : ____   Hunger rating before eating ____   Hunger rating after eating ____

Snack   ____ : ____   Hunger rating before eating ____   Hunger rating after eating ____

Other meal/snack   ____ : ____   Hunger rating before eating ____   Hunger rating after eating ____

Other meal/snack   ____ : ____   Hunger rating before eating ____   Hunger rating after eating ____

Did you meet your hunger scale goals?   Y   N

NOTES _____

_____

Write down the number of servings you had in each food group. For Anything Goes, just write down the total number of treat calories you had. For a refresher on what counts as a serving, see page 119 in *The Best Life Diet*. And to find out how many servings of grains, fruit, and the other food groups you should have daily (and how many Anything Goes Calories you get), look at the chart on page 119 of the book. (Remember, you can also track your intake and get feedback by joining www.thebestlife.com.)

	Breakfast	Lunch	Dinner	Snack	Other	Other
Grain/Starchy Vegetables						
Fruit						
Vegetables						
Dairy (preferably nonfat or 1%)						
Protein-Rich Foods						
Fat (preferably healthy)						
Anything Goes Calories						

Are your portions becoming more reasonable?   Y   N

NOTES _____

_____

Did you stay within your Anything Goes Calories for treats?   Y   N

NOTES _____

_____

_____

_____

_____

_____

_____

_____

_____

_____

_____

_____

_____

_____

_____

_____

_____

_____

ACTIVITY LEVEL: 0   1   2   3   4   5

Aerobic minutes or steps/day _____

Did you meet your aerobic/step goal?   Y   N

NOTES _____

_____

STRENGTH TRAINING

Exercise								
Weight								
Reps								
Sets								

Did you meet your strength-training goal?   Y   N

NOTES _____

_____

Eating cutoff time: ____ : ____   Bedtime: ____ : ____

Did you cut off eating at least two hours before bedtime?   Y   N

Did you eat three meals (including a nutritious breakfast) and at least one snack?   Y   N

Did you eliminate the six problem foods from your diet?   Y   N

Did you drink at least six 8-ounce glasses of water?   Y   N

Did you take your vitamin supplements?   Y   N

                    TIME

Breakfast   ____ : ____   Hunger rating before eating ____   Hunger rating after eating ____

Lunch   ____ : ____   Hunger rating before eating ____   Hunger rating after eating ____

Dinner   ____ : ____   Hunger rating before eating ____   Hunger rating after eating ____

Snack   ____ : ____   Hunger rating before eating ____   Hunger rating after eating ____

Other meal/snack ____ : ____   Hunger rating before eating ____   Hunger rating after eating ____

Other meal/snack ____ : ____   Hunger rating before eating ____   Hunger rating after eating ____

Did you meet your hunger scale goals?   Y   N

NOTES _____

_____

Write down the number of servings you had in each food group. For Anything Goes, just write down the total number of treat calories you had. For a refresher on what counts as a serving, see page 119 in *The Best Life Diet*. And to find out how many servings of grains, fruit, and the other food groups you should have daily (and how many Anything Goes Calories you get), look at the chart on page 119 of the book. (Remember, you can also track your intake and get feedback by joining www.thebestlife.com.)

	Breakfast	Lunch	Dinner	Snack	Other	Other
Grain/Starchy Vegetables						
Fruit						
Vegetables						
Dairy (preferably nonfat or 1%)						
Protein-Rich Foods						
Fat (preferably healthy)						
Anything Goes Calories						

Are your portions becoming more reasonable?   Y   N

NOTES _____

_____

Did you stay within your Anything Goes Calories for treats?   Y   N

NOTES _____

_____

_____

_____

_____

_____

_____

_____

_____

_____

_____

_____

_____

_____

_____

_____

_____

_____

ACTIVITY LEVEL: 0   1   2   3   4   5

Aerobic minutes or steps/day _____

Did you meet your aerobic/step goal?   Y   N

NOTES _____

_____

STRENGTH TRAINING

Exercise								
Weight								
Reps								
Sets								

Did you meet your strength-training goal?   Y   N

NOTES _____

_____

Eating cutoff time: _____:_____   Bedtime: _____:_____

Did you cut off eating at least two hours before bedtime?   Y   N

Did you eat three meals (including a nutritious breakfast) and at least one snack?   Y   N

Did you eliminate the six problem foods from your diet?   Y   N

Did you drink at least six 8-ounce glasses of water?   Y   N

Did you take your vitamin supplements?   Y   N

TIME

Breakfast _____:_____ Hunger rating before eating _____ Hunger rating after eating _____

Lunch _____:_____ Hunger rating before eating _____ Hunger rating after eating _____

Dinner _____:_____ Hunger rating before eating _____ Hunger rating after eating _____

Snack _____:_____ Hunger rating before eating _____ Hunger rating after eating _____

Other meal/snack _____:_____ Hunger rating before eating _____ Hunger rating after eating _____

Other meal/snack _____:_____ Hunger rating before eating _____ Hunger rating after eating _____

Did you meet your hunger scale goals?   Y   N

NOTES _____

_____

Write down the number of servings you had in each food group. For Anything Goes, just write down the total number of treat calories you had. For a refresher on what counts as a serving, see page 119 in *The Best Life Diet*. And to find out how many servings of grains, fruit, and the other food groups you should have daily (and how many Anything Goes Calories you get), look at the chart on page 119 of the book. (Remember, you can also track your intake and get feedback by joining www.thebestlife.com.)

	Breakfast	Lunch	Dinner	Snack	Other	Other
Grain/Starchy Vegetables						
Fruit						
Vegetables						
Dairy (preferably nonfat or 1%)						
Protein-Rich Foods						
Fat (preferably healthy)						
Anything Goes Calories						

Are your portions becoming more reasonable?   Y   N

NOTES _____

_____

Did you stay within your Anything Goes Calories for treats?   Y   N

NOTES _____

_____

_____

_____

_____

_____

_____

_____

_____

_____

_____

_____

_____

_____

_____

_____

_____

_____

ACTIVITY LEVEL: 0   1   2   3   4   5

Aerobic minutes or steps/day _____

Did you meet your aerobic/step goal?   Y   N

NOTES _____

STRENGTH TRAINING

Exercise								
Weight								
Reps								
Sets								

Did you meet your strength-training goal?   Y   N

NOTES _____

Eating cutoff time: ____:____   Bedtime: ____:____

Did you cut off eating at least two hours before bedtime?   Y   N

Did you eat three meals (including a nutritious breakfast) and at least one snack?   Y   N

Did you eliminate the six problem foods from your diet?   Y   N

Did you drink at least six 8-ounce glasses of water?   Y   N

Did you take your vitamin supplements?   Y   N

                     TIME

Breakfast   ____:____   Hunger rating before eating _____   Hunger rating after eating _____

Lunch   ____:____   Hunger rating before eating _____   Hunger rating after eating _____

Dinner   ____:____   Hunger rating before eating _____   Hunger rating after eating _____

Snack   ____:____   Hunger rating before eating _____   Hunger rating after eating _____

Other meal/snack   ____:____   Hunger rating before eating _____   Hunger rating after eating _____

Other meal/snack   ____:____   Hunger rating before eating _____   Hunger rating after eating _____

Did you meet your hunger scale goals?   Y   N

NOTES _____
_____

Write down the number of servings you had in each food group. For Anything Goes, just write down the total number of treat calories you had. For a refresher on what counts as a serving, see page 119 in *The Best Life Diet*. And to find out how many servings of grains, fruit, and the other food groups you should have daily (and how many Anything Goes Calories you get), look at the chart on page 119 of the book. (Remember, you can also track your intake and get feedback by joining www.thebestlife.com.)

	Breakfast	Lunch	Dinner	Snack	Other	Other
Grain/Starchy Vegetables						
Fruit						
Vegetables						
Dairy (preferably nonfat or 1%)						
Protein-Rich Foods						
Fat (preferably healthy)						
Anything Goes Calories						

Are your portions becoming more reasonable?   Y   N
NOTES _____
_____

Did you stay within your Anything Goes Calories for treats?   Y   N
NOTES _____
_____
_____
_____
_____
_____
_____
_____
_____
_____
_____
_____
_____
_____
_____
_____
_____

WEEK: DATE: PHASE 2

ACTIVITY LEVEL: 0 1 2 3 4 5

Aerobic minutes or steps/day _____

Did you meet your aerobic/step goal? Y N

NOTES _____

STRENGTH TRAINING

Exercise								
Weight								
Reps								
Sets								

Did you meet your strength-training goal? Y N

NOTES _____

Eating cutoff time: _____:_____   Bedtime: _____:_____

Did you cut off eating at least two hours before bedtime? Y N

Did you eat three meals (including a nutritious breakfast) and at least one snack? Y N

Did you eliminate the six problem foods from your diet? Y N

Did you drink at least six 8-ounce glasses of water? Y N

Did you take your vitamin supplements? Y N

TIME

Breakfast _____:_____ Hunger rating before eating _____ Hunger rating after eating _____

Lunch _____:_____ Hunger rating before eating _____ Hunger rating after eating _____

Dinner _____:_____ Hunger rating before eating _____ Hunger rating after eating _____

Snack _____:_____ Hunger rating before eating _____ Hunger rating after eating _____

Other meal/snack _____:_____ Hunger rating before eating _____ Hunger rating after eating _____

Other meal/snack _____:_____ Hunger rating before eating _____ Hunger rating after eating _____

Did you meet your hunger scale goals? Y N

NOTES _____

Write down the number of servings you had in each food group. For Anything Goes, just write down the total number of treat calories you had. For a refresher on what counts as a serving, see page 119 in *The Best Life Diet*. And to find out how many servings of grains, fruit, and the other food groups you should have daily (and how many Anything Goes Calories you get), look at the chart on page 119 of the book. (Remember, you can also track your intake and get feedback by joining www.thebestlife.com.)

	Breakfast	Lunch	Dinner	Snack	Other	Other
Grain/Starchy Vegetables						
Fruit						
Vegetables						
Dairy (preferably nonfat or 1%)						
Protein-Rich Foods						
Fat (preferably healthy)						
Anything Goes Calories						

Are your portions becoming more reasonable?   Y   N

NOTES _____

_____

Did you stay within your Anything Goes Calories for treats?   Y   N

NOTES _____

_____

_____

_____

_____

_____

_____

_____

_____

_____

_____

_____

_____

_____

_____

_____

_____

Weekly Summary

WEEK: _____   PHASE 2

Your weight: _____

Total aerobic minutes/steps for the week _____

Did you meet your aerobic/step goal?   Y   N

Did you meet your strength-training goals for the week?   Y   N

How many days did you cut off your eating at least two hours before bedtime? _____

How many days did you eat three meals and at least one snack? _____

How many days did eliminate the six problem foods? _____

How many days did you drink at least six 8-ounce glasses of water? _____

How many days did you take your vitamin supplements? _____

How many days did you meet your hunger scale goals? _____

How many days did you eat reasonable portions? _____

How many days did you stay within your Anything Goes Calories for treats? _____

How was your week overall? _____

_____

_____

_____

_____

_____

_____

_____

_____

_____

_____

_____

_____

_____

_____

_____

ACTIVITY LEVEL: 0 1 2 3 4 5

Aerobic minutes or steps/day _____

Did you meet your aerobic/step goal?   Y   N

NOTES _____

STRENGTH TRAINING

Exercise								
Weight								
Reps								
Sets								

Did you meet your strength-training goal?   Y   N

NOTES _____

Eating cutoff time: ___ : ___   Bedtime: ___ : ___

Did you cut off eating at least two hours before bedtime?   Y   N

Did you eat three meals (including a nutritious breakfast) and at least one snack?   Y   N

Did you eliminate the six problem foods from your diet?   Y   N

Did you drink at least six 8-ounce glasses of water?   Y   N

Did you take your vitamin supplements?   Y   N

         TIME

Breakfast   ___ : ___   Hunger rating before eating ___   Hunger rating after eating ___

Lunch   ___ : ___   Hunger rating before eating ___   Hunger rating after eating ___

Dinner   ___ : ___   Hunger rating before eating ___   Hunger rating after eating ___

Snack   ___ : ___   Hunger rating before eating ___   Hunger rating after eating ___

Other meal/snack ___ : ___   Hunger rating before eating ___   Hunger rating after eating ___

Other meal/snack ___ : ___   Hunger rating before eating ___   Hunger rating after eating ___

Did you meet your hunger scale goals?   Y   N

NOTES _____

Write down the number of servings you had in each food group. For Anything Goes, just write down the total number of treat calories you had. For a refresher on what counts as a serving, see page 119 in *The Best Life Diet*. And to find out how many servings of grains, fruit, and the other food groups you should have daily (and how many Anything Goes Calories you get), look at the chart on page 119 of the book. (Remember, you can also track your intake and get feedback by joining www.thebestlife.com.)

	Breakfast	Lunch	Dinner	Snack	Other	Other
Grain/Starchy Vegetables						
Fruit						
Vegetables						
Dairy (preferably nonfat or 1%)						
Protein-Rich Foods						
Fat (preferably healthy)						
Anything Goes Calories						

Are your portions becoming more reasonable?   Y   N

NOTES _____

_____

Did you stay within your Anything Goes Calories for treats?   Y   N

NOTES _____

_____

_____

_____

_____

_____

_____

_____

_____

_____

_____

_____

_____

_____

_____

_____

_____

_____

ACTIVITY LEVEL: 0   1   2   3   4   5

Aerobic minutes or steps/day _____

Did you meet your aerobic/step goal?   Y   N

NOTES _____

_____

STRENGTH TRAINING

Exercise								
Weight								
Reps								
Sets								

Did you meet your strength-training goal?   Y   N

NOTES _____

_____

Eating cutoff time: ____:____   Bedtime: ____:____

Did you cut off eating at least two hours before bedtime?   Y   N

Did you eat three meals (including a nutritious breakfast) and at least one snack?   Y   N

Did you eliminate the six problem foods from your diet?   Y   N

Did you drink at least six 8-ounce glasses of water?   Y   N

Did you take your vitamin supplements?   Y   N

	TIME		
Breakfast	____:____	Hunger rating before eating ____	Hunger rating after eating ____
Lunch	____:____	Hunger rating before eating ____	Hunger rating after eating ____
Dinner	____:____	Hunger rating before eating ____	Hunger rating after eating ____
Snack	____:____	Hunger rating before eating ____	Hunger rating after eating ____
Other meal/snack	____:____	Hunger rating before eating ____	Hunger rating after eating ____
Other meal/snack	____:____	Hunger rating before eating ____	Hunger rating after eating ____

Did you meet your hunger scale goals?   Y   N

NOTES _____

_____

Write down the number of servings you had in each food group. For Anything Goes, just write down the total number of treat calories you had. For a refresher on what counts as a serving, see page 119 in *The Best Life Diet*. And to find out how many servings of grains, fruit, and the other food groups you should have daily (and how many Anything Goes Calories you get), look at the chart on page 119 of the book. (Remember, you can also track your intake and get feedback by joining www.thebestlife.com.)

	Breakfast	Lunch	Dinner	Snack	Other	Other
Grain/Starchy Vegetables						
Fruit						
Vegetables						
Dairy (preferably nonfat or 1%)						
Protein-Rich Foods						
Fat (preferably healthy)						
Anything Goes Calories						

Are your portions becoming more reasonable?   Y   N

NOTES _____

_____

Did you stay within your Anything Goes Calories for treats?   Y   N

NOTES _____

_____

_____

_____

_____

_____

_____

_____

_____

_____

_____

_____

_____

_____

_____

_____

_____

ACTIVITY LEVEL: 0   1   2   3   4   5

Aerobic minutes or steps/day _____

Did you meet your aerobic/step goal?   Y   N

NOTES _____

_____

STRENGTH TRAINING

Exercise								
Weight								
Reps								
Sets								

Did you meet your strength-training goal?   Y   N

NOTES _____

_____

Eating cutoff time: ____ : ____   Bedtime: ____ : ____

Did you cut off eating at least two hours before bedtime?   Y   N

Did you eat three meals (including a nutritious breakfast) and at least one snack?   Y   N

Did you eliminate the six problem foods from your diet?   Y   N

Did you drink at least six 8-ounce glasses of water?   Y   N

Did you take your vitamin supplements?   Y   N

                  TIME

Breakfast   ____ : ____   Hunger rating before eating ____   Hunger rating after eating ____

Lunch   ____ : ____   Hunger rating before eating ____   Hunger rating after eating ____

Dinner   ____ : ____   Hunger rating before eating ____   Hunger rating after eating ____

Snack   ____ : ____   Hunger rating before eating ____   Hunger rating after eating ____

Other meal/snack   ____ : ____   Hunger rating before eating ____   Hunger rating after eating ____

Other meal/snack   ____ : ____   Hunger rating before eating ____   Hunger rating after eating ____

Did you meet your hunger scale goals?   Y   N

NOTES _____

_____

Write down the number of servings you had in each food group. For Anything Goes, just write down the total number of treat calories you had. For a refresher on what counts as a serving, see page 119 in *The Best Life Diet*. And to find out how many servings of grains, fruit, and the other food groups you should have daily (and how many Anything Goes Calories you get), look at the chart on page 119 of the book. (Remember, you can also track your intake and get feedback by joining www.thebestlife.com.)

	Breakfast	Lunch	Dinner	Snack	Other	Other
Grain/Starchy Vegetables						
Fruit						
Vegetables						
Dairy (preferably nonfat or 1%)						
Protein-Rich Foods						
Fat (preferably healthy)						
Anything Goes Calories						

Are your portions becoming more reasonable? Y N

NOTES _____

_____

Did you stay within your Anything Goes Calories for treats? Y N

NOTES _____

_____

_____

_____

_____

_____

_____

_____

_____

_____

_____

_____

_____

_____

_____

_____

_____

_____

WEEK: DATE:
PHASE 2

ACTIVITY LEVEL: 0 1 2 3 4 5

Aerobic minutes or steps/day _____

Did you meet your aerobic/step goal? Y N

NOTES _____

STRENGTH TRAINING

Exercise								
Weight								
Reps								
Sets								

Did you meet your strength-training goal? Y N

NOTES _____

Eating cutoff time: _____ : _____ Bedtime: _____ : _____

Did you cut off eating at least two hours before bedtime? Y N

Did you eat three meals (including a nutritious breakfast) and at least one snack? Y N

Did you eliminate the six problem foods from your diet? Y N

Did you drink at least six 8-ounce glasses of water? Y N

Did you take your vitamin supplements? Y N

TIME

Breakfast	_____ : _____	Hunger rating before eating _____	Hunger rating after eating _____
Lunch	_____ : _____	Hunger rating before eating _____	Hunger rating after eating _____
Dinner	_____ : _____	Hunger rating before eating _____	Hunger rating after eating _____
Snack	_____ : _____	Hunger rating before eating _____	Hunger rating after eating _____
Other meal/snack	_____ : _____	Hunger rating before eating _____	Hunger rating after eating _____
Other meal/snack	_____ : _____	Hunger rating before eating _____	Hunger rating after eating _____

Did you meet your hunger scale goals? Y N

NOTES _____

_____

Write down the number of servings you had in each food group. For Anything Goes, just write down the total number of treat calories you had. For a refresher on what counts as a serving, see page 119 in *The Best Life Diet*. And to find out how many servings of grains, fruit, and the other food groups you should have daily (and how many Anything Goes Calories you get), look at the chart on page 119 of the book. (Remember, you can also track your intake and get feedback by joining www.thebestlife.com.)

	Breakfast	Lunch	Dinner	Snack	Other	Other
Grain/Starchy Vegetables						
Fruit						
Vegetables						
Dairy (preferably nonfat or 1%)						
Protein-Rich Foods						
Fat (preferably healthy)						
Anything Goes Calories						

Are your portions becoming more reasonable?   Y   N

NOTES _____

_____

Did you stay within your Anything Goes Calories for treats?   Y   N

NOTES _____

_____

_____

_____

_____

_____

_____

_____

_____

_____

_____

_____

_____

_____

_____

_____

_____

_____

ACTIVITY LEVEL: 0 1 2 3 4 5

Aerobic minutes or steps/day _____

Did you meet your aerobic/step goal? Y N

NOTES _____

STRENGTH TRAINING

Exercise								
Weight								
Reps								
Sets								

Did you meet your strength-training goal? Y N

NOTES _____

Eating cutoff time: ____ : ____   Bedtime: ____ : ____

Did you cut off eating at least two hours before bedtime? Y N

Did you eat three meals (including a nutritious breakfast) and at least one snack? Y N

Did you eliminate the six problem foods from your diet? Y N

Did you drink at least six 8-ounce glasses of water? Y N

Did you take your vitamin supplements? Y N

TIME

Breakfast ____ : ____ Hunger rating before eating ____ Hunger rating after eating ____

Lunch ____ : ____ Hunger rating before eating ____ Hunger rating after eating ____

Dinner ____ : ____ Hunger rating before eating ____ Hunger rating after eating ____

Snack ____ : ____ Hunger rating before eating ____ Hunger rating after eating ____

Other meal/snack ____ : ____ Hunger rating before eating ____ Hunger rating after eating ____

Other meal/snack ____ : ____ Hunger rating before eating ____ Hunger rating after eating ____

Did you meet your hunger scale goals? Y N

NOTES _____

Write down the number of servings you had in each food group. For Anything Goes, just write down the total number of treat calories you had. For a refresher on what counts as a serving, see page 119 in *The Best Life Diet*. And to find out how many servings of grains, fruit, and the other food groups you should have daily (and how many Anything Goes Calories you get), look at the chart on page 119 of the book. (Remember, you can also track your intake and get feedback by joining www.thebestlife.com.)

	Breakfast	Lunch	Dinner	Snack	Other	Other
Grain/Starchy Vegetables						
Fruit						
Vegetables						
Dairy (preferably nonfat or 1%)						
Protein-Rich Foods						
Fat (preferably healthy)						
Anything Goes Calories						

Are your portions becoming more reasonable? Y N

NOTES _____

_____

Did you stay within your Anything Goes Calories for treats? Y N

NOTES _____

_____

_____

_____

_____

_____

_____

_____

_____

_____

_____

_____

_____

_____

_____

_____

_____

_____

_____

_____

ACTIVITY LEVEL: 0 1 2 3 4 5

Aerobic minutes or steps/day _____

Did you meet your aerobic/step goal? Y N

NOTES _____

_____

STRENGTH TRAINING

Exercise								
Weight								
Reps								
Sets								

Did you meet your strength-training goal? Y N

NOTES _____

_____

Eating cutoff time: ___ : ___   Bedtime: ___ : ___

Did you cut off eating at least two hours before bedtime? Y N

Did you eat three meals (including a nutritious breakfast) and at least one snack? Y N

Did you eliminate the six problem foods from your diet? Y N

Did you drink at least six 8-ounce glasses of water? Y N

Did you take your vitamin supplements? Y N

TIME

Breakfast ___ : ___ Hunger rating before eating ___ Hunger rating after eating ___

Lunch ___ : ___ Hunger rating before eating ___ Hunger rating after eating ___

Dinner ___ : ___ Hunger rating before eating ___ Hunger rating after eating ___

Snack ___ : ___ Hunger rating before eating ___ Hunger rating after eating ___

Other meal/snack ___ : ___ Hunger rating before eating ___ Hunger rating after eating ___

Other meal/snack ___ : ___ Hunger rating before eating ___ Hunger rating after eating ___

Did you meet your hunger scale goals? Y N

NOTES _____

_____

Write down the number of servings you had in each food group. For Anything Goes, just write down the total number of treat calories you had. For a refresher on what counts as a serving, see page 119 in *The Best Life Diet*. And to find out how many servings of grains, fruit, and the other food groups you should have daily (and how many Anything Goes Calories you get), look at the chart on page 119 of the book. (Remember, you can also track your intake and get feedback by joining www.thebestlife.com.)

	Breakfast	Lunch	Dinner	Snack	Other	Other
Grain/Starchy Vegetables						
Fruit						
Vegetables						
Dairy (preferably nonfat or 1%)						
Protein-Rich Foods						
Fat (preferably healthy)						
Anything Goes Calories						

Are your portions becoming more reasonable?   Y   N

NOTES _____

_____

Did you stay within your Anything Goes Calories for treats?   Y   N

NOTES _____

_____

_____

_____

_____

_____

_____

_____

_____

_____

_____

_____

_____

_____

_____

_____

_____

_____

_____

ACTIVITY LEVEL: 0   1   2   3   4   5

Aerobic minutes or steps/day _____

Did you meet your aerobic/step goal?   Y   N

NOTES _____

STRENGTH TRAINING

Exercise								
Weight								
Reps								
Sets								

Did you meet your strength-training goal?   Y   N

NOTES _____

Eating cutoff time: ____ : ____   Bedtime: ____ : ____

Did you cut off eating at least two hours before bedtime?   Y   N

Did you eat three meals (including a nutritious breakfast) and at least one snack?   Y   N

Did you eliminate the six problem foods from your diet?   Y   N

Did you drink at least six 8-ounce glasses of water?   Y   N

Did you take your vitamin supplements?   Y   N

                  TIME

Breakfast   ____ : ____   Hunger rating before eating ____   Hunger rating after eating ____

Lunch   ____ : ____   Hunger rating before eating ____   Hunger rating after eating ____

Dinner   ____ : ____   Hunger rating before eating ____   Hunger rating after eating ____

Snack   ____ : ____   Hunger rating before eating ____   Hunger rating after eating ____

Other meal/snack ____ : ____   Hunger rating before eating ____   Hunger rating after eating ____

Other meal/snack ____ : ____   Hunger rating before eating ____   Hunger rating after eating ____

Did you meet your hunger scale goals?   Y   N

NOTES _____

_____

Write down the number of servings you had in each food group. For Anything Goes, just write down the total number of treat calories you had. For a refresher on what counts as a serving, see page 119 in *The Best Life Diet*. And to find out how many servings of grains, fruit, and the other food groups you should have daily (and how many Anything Goes Calories you get), look at the chart on page 119 of the book. (Remember, you can also track your intake and get feedback by joining www.thebestlife.com.)

	Breakfast	Lunch	Dinner	Snack	Other	Other
Grain/Starchy Vegetables						
Fruit						
Vegetables						
Dairy (preferably nonfat or 1%)						
Protein-Rich Foods						
Fat (preferably healthy)						
Anything Goes Calories						

Are your portions becoming more reasonable?   Y   N

NOTES _____

_____

Did you stay within your Anything Goes Calories for treats?   Y   N

NOTES _____

_____

_____

_____

_____

_____

_____

_____

_____

_____

_____

_____

_____

_____

_____

_____

_____

_____

Weekly Summary

Your weight: _____

Total aerobic minutes/steps for the week _____

Did you meet your aerobic/step goal?   Y   N

Did you meet your strength-training goals for the week?   Y   N

How many days did you cut off your eating at least two hours before bedtime? _____

How many days did you eat three meals and at least one snack? _____

How many days did eliminate the six problem foods? _____

How many days did you drink at least six 8-ounce glasses of water? _____

How many days did you take your vitamin supplements? _____

How many days did you meet your hunger scale goals? _____

How many days did you eat reasonable portions? _____

How many days did you stay within your Anything Goes Calories for treats? _____

How was your week overall? _____

ACTIVITY LEVEL: 0   1   2   3   4   5

Aerobic minutes or steps/day _____

Did you meet your aerobic/step goal?   Y   N

NOTES _____

STRENGTH TRAINING

Exercise								
Weight								
Reps								
Sets								

Did you meet your strength-training goal?   Y   N

NOTES _____

Eating cutoff time: _____ : _____   Bedtime: _____ : _____

Did you cut off eating at least two hours before bedtime?   Y   N

Did you eat three meals (including a nutritious breakfast) and at least one snack?   Y   N

Did you eliminate the six problem foods from your diet?   Y   N

Did you drink at least six 8-ounce glasses of water?   Y   N

Did you take your vitamin supplements?   Y   N

                     TIME

Breakfast   _____ : _____   Hunger rating before eating _____ Hunger rating after eating _____

Lunch   _____ : _____   Hunger rating before eating _____ Hunger rating after eating _____

Dinner   _____ : _____   Hunger rating before eating _____ Hunger rating after eating _____

Snack   _____ : _____   Hunger rating before eating _____ Hunger rating after eating _____

Other meal/snack _____ : _____   Hunger rating before eating _____ Hunger rating after eating _____

Other meal/snack _____ : _____   Hunger rating before eating _____ Hunger rating after eating _____

Did you meet your hunger scale goals?   Y   N

NOTES _____

Write down the number of servings you had in each food group. For Anything Goes, just write down the total number of treat calories you had. For a refresher on what counts as a serving, see page 119 in *The Best Life Diet*. And to find out how many servings of grains, fruit, and the other food groups you should have daily (and how many Anything Goes Calories you get), look at the chart on page 119 of the book. (Remember, you can also track your intake and get feedback by joining www.thebestlife.com.)

	Breakfast	Lunch	Dinner	Snack	Other	Other
Grain/Starchy Vegetables						
Fruit						
Vegetables						
Dairy (preferably nonfat or 1%)						
Protein-Rich Foods						
Fat (preferably healthy)						
Anything Goes Calories						

Are your portions becoming more reasonable?   Y   N

NOTES _____

_____

Did you stay within your Anything Goes Calories for treats?   Y   N

NOTES _____

_____

_____

_____

_____

_____

_____

_____

_____

_____

_____

_____

_____

_____

_____

_____

_____

_____

_____

_____

WEEK: **DATE:**   **PHASE 2**

ACTIVITY LEVEL: 0   1   2   3   4   5

Aerobic minutes or steps/day _____

Did you meet your aerobic/step goal?   Y   N

NOTES _____

_____

STRENGTH TRAINING

Exercise								
Weight								
Reps								
Sets								

Did you meet your strength-training goal?   Y   N

NOTES _____

_____

Eating cutoff time: _____ : _____   Bedtime: _____ : _____

Did you cut off eating at least two hours before bedtime?   Y   N

Did you eat three meals (including a nutritious breakfast) and at least one snack?   Y   N

Did you eliminate the six problem foods from your diet?   Y   N

Did you drink at least six 8-ounce glasses of water?   Y   N

Did you take your vitamin supplements?   Y   N

                     TIME

Breakfast   _____ : _____   Hunger rating before eating _____   Hunger rating after eating _____

Lunch   _____ : _____   Hunger rating before eating _____   Hunger rating after eating _____

Dinner   _____ : _____   Hunger rating before eating _____   Hunger rating after eating _____

Snack   _____ : _____   Hunger rating before eating _____   Hunger rating after eating _____

Other meal/snack _____ : _____   Hunger rating before eating _____   Hunger rating after eating _____

Other meal/snack _____ : _____   Hunger rating before eating _____   Hunger rating after eating _____

Did you meet your hunger scale goals?   Y   N

NOTES _____

_____

Write down the number of servings you had in each food group. For Anything Goes, just write down the total number of treat calories you had. For a refresher on what counts as a serving, see page 119 in *The Best Life Diet*. And to find out how many servings of grains, fruit, and the other food groups you should have daily (and how many Anything Goes Calories you get), look at the chart on page 119 of the book. (Remember, you can also track your intake and get feedback by joining www.thebestlife.com.)

	Breakfast	Lunch	Dinner	Snack	Other	Other
Grain/Starchy Vegetables						
Fruit						
Vegetables						
Dairy (preferably nonfat or 1%)						
Protein-Rich Foods						
Fat (preferably healthy)						
Anything Goes Calories						

Are your portions becoming more reasonable?　　　　　　　　　　　　　　　Y　N

NOTES _____

_____

Did you stay within your Anything Goes Calories for treats?　　　　　　　Y　N

NOTES _____

_____

_____

_____

_____

_____

_____

_____

_____

_____

_____

_____

_____

_____

_____

_____

_____

_____

ACTIVITY LEVEL: 0 1 2 3 4 5

Aerobic minutes or steps/day _____

Did you meet your aerobic/step goal?   Y   N

NOTES _____

_____

STRENGTH TRAINING

Exercise								
Weight								
Reps								
Sets								

Did you meet your strength-training goal?   Y   N

NOTES _____

_____

Eating cutoff time: ____:____   Bedtime: ____:____

Did you cut off eating at least two hours before bedtime?   Y   N

Did you eat three meals (including a nutritious breakfast) and at least one snack?   Y   N

Did you eliminate the six problem foods from your diet?   Y   N

Did you drink at least six 8-ounce glasses of water?   Y   N

Did you take your vitamin supplements?   Y   N

               TIME

Breakfast   ____:____   Hunger rating before eating ____   Hunger rating after eating ____

Lunch   ____:____   Hunger rating before eating ____   Hunger rating after eating ____

Dinner   ____:____   Hunger rating before eating ____   Hunger rating after eating ____

Snack   ____:____   Hunger rating before eating ____   Hunger rating after eating ____

Other meal/snack   ____:____   Hunger rating before eating ____   Hunger rating after eating ____

Other meal/snack   ____:____   Hunger rating before eating ____   Hunger rating after eating ____

Did you meet your hunger scale goals?   Y   N

NOTES _____

_____

Write down the number of servings you had in each food group. For Anything Goes, just write down the total number of treat calories you had. For a refresher on what counts as a serving, see page 119 in *The Best Life Diet*. And to find out how many servings of grains, fruit, and the other food groups you should have daily (and how many Anything Goes Calories you get), look at the chart on page 119 of the book. (Remember, you can also track your intake and get feedback by joining www.thebestlife.com.)

	Breakfast	Lunch	Dinner	Snack	Other	Other
Grain/Starchy Vegetables						
Fruit						
Vegetables						
Dairy (preferably nonfat or 1%)						
Protein-Rich Foods						
Fat (preferably healthy)						
Anything Goes Calories						

Are your portions becoming more reasonable?　　　　　　　　　　　　　　Y　N

NOTES _____

_____

Did you stay within your Anything Goes Calories for treats?　　　　　　Y　N

NOTES _____

_____

_____

_____

_____

_____

_____

_____

_____

_____

_____

_____

_____

_____

_____

_____

_____

_____

ACTIVITY LEVEL: 0   1   2   3   4   5

Aerobic minutes or steps/day _____

Did you meet your aerobic/step goal?   Y   N
NOTES _____

STRENGTH TRAINING

Exercise								
Weight								
Reps								
Sets								

Did you meet your strength-training goal?   Y   N
NOTES _____

Eating cutoff time: ____ : _____   Bedtime: ____ : _____

Did you cut off eating at least two hours before bedtime?   Y   N

Did you eat three meals (including a nutritious breakfast) and at least one snack?   Y   N

Did you eliminate the six problem foods from your diet?   Y   N

Did you drink at least six 8-ounce glasses of water?   Y   N

Did you take your vitamin supplements?   Y   N

	TIME		
Breakfast	____ : _____	Hunger rating before eating _____	Hunger rating after eating _____
Lunch	____ : _____	Hunger rating before eating _____	Hunger rating after eating _____
Dinner	____ : _____	Hunger rating before eating _____	Hunger rating after eating _____
Snack	____ : _____	Hunger rating before eating _____	Hunger rating after eating _____
Other meal/snack	____ : _____	Hunger rating before eating _____	Hunger rating after eating _____
Other meal/snack	____ : _____	Hunger rating before eating _____	Hunger rating after eating _____

Did you meet your hunger scale goals?   Y   N
NOTES _____
_____

Write down the number of servings you had in each food group. For Anything Goes, just write down the total number of treat calories you had. For a refresher on what counts as a serving, see page 119 in *The Best Life Diet*. And to find out how many servings of grains, fruit, and the other food groups you should have daily (and how many Anything Goes Calories you get), look at the chart on page 119 of the book. (Remember, you can also track your intake and get feedback by joining www.thebestlife.com.)

	Breakfast	Lunch	Dinner	Snack	Other	Other
Grain/Starchy Vegetables						
Fruit						
Vegetables						
Dairy (preferably nonfat or 1%)						
Protein-Rich Foods						
Fat (preferably healthy)						
Anything Goes Calories						

Are your portions becoming more reasonable?   Y   N

NOTES _____

_____

Did you stay within your Anything Goes Calories for treats?   Y   N

NOTES _____

_____

_____

_____

_____

_____

_____

_____

_____

_____

_____

_____

_____

_____

_____

_____

_____

ACTIVITY LEVEL: 0   1   2   3   4   5

Aerobic minutes or steps/day _____

Did you meet your aerobic/step goal?   Y   N

NOTES _____

STRENGTH TRAINING

Exercise								
Weight								
Reps								
Sets								

Did you meet your strength-training goal?   Y   N

NOTES _____

Eating cutoff time: ____ : ____   Bedtime: ____ : ____

Did you cut off eating at least two hours before bedtime?   Y   N

Did you eat three meals (including a nutritious breakfast) and at least one snack?   Y   N

Did you eliminate the six problem foods from your diet?   Y   N

Did you drink at least six 8-ounce glasses of water?   Y   N

Did you take your vitamin supplements?   Y   N

                     TIME

Breakfast   ____ : ____   Hunger rating before eating ____   Hunger rating after eating ____

Lunch   ____ : ____   Hunger rating before eating ____   Hunger rating after eating ____

Dinner   ____ : ____   Hunger rating before eating ____   Hunger rating after eating ____

Snack   ____ : ____   Hunger rating before eating ____   Hunger rating after eating ____

Other meal/snack   ____ : ____   Hunger rating before eating ____   Hunger rating after eating ____

Other meal/snack   ____ : ____   Hunger rating before eating ____   Hunger rating after eating ____

Did you meet your hunger scale goals?   Y   N

NOTES _____

Write down the number of servings you had in each food group. For Anything Goes, just write down the total number of treat calories you had. For a refresher on what counts as a serving, see page 119 in *The Best Life Diet*. And to find out how many servings of grains, fruit, and the other food groups you should have daily (and how many Anything Goes Calories you get), look at the chart on page 119 of the book. (Remember, you can also track your intake and get feedback by joining www.thebestlife.com.)

	Breakfast	Lunch	Dinner	Snack	Other	Other
Grain/Starchy Vegetables						
Fruit						
Vegetables						
Dairy (preferably nonfat or 1%)						
Protein-Rich Foods						
Fat (preferably healthy)						
Anything Goes Calories						

Are your portions becoming more reasonable?　　　　　　　　　　　　　　　Y　N

NOTES _____

_____

Did you stay within your Anything Goes Calories for treats?　　　　　　　　Y　N

NOTES _____

_____

_____

_____

_____

_____

_____

_____

_____

_____

_____

_____

_____

_____

_____

_____

_____

_____

_____

_____

ACTIVITY LEVEL: 0   1   2   3   4   5

Aerobic minutes or steps/day _____

Did you meet your aerobic/step goal?   Y   N

NOTES _____

STRENGTH TRAINING

Exercise								
Weight								
Reps								
Sets								

Did you meet your strength-training goal?   Y   N

NOTES _____

Eating cutoff time: ____:____   Bedtime: ____:____

Did you cut off eating at least two hours before bedtime?   Y   N

Did you eat three meals (including a nutritious breakfast) and at least one snack?   Y   N

Did you eliminate the six problem foods from your diet?   Y   N

Did you drink at least six 8-ounce glasses of water?   Y   N

Did you take your vitamin supplements?   Y   N

                     TIME

Breakfast   ____:____   Hunger rating before eating _____ Hunger rating after eating _____

Lunch   ____:____   Hunger rating before eating _____ Hunger rating after eating _____

Dinner   ____:____   Hunger rating before eating _____ Hunger rating after eating _____

Snack   ____:____   Hunger rating before eating _____ Hunger rating after eating _____

Other meal/snack ____:____   Hunger rating before eating _____ Hunger rating after eating _____

Other meal/snack ____:____   Hunger rating before eating _____ Hunger rating after eating _____

Did you meet your hunger scale goals?   Y   N

NOTES _____

_____

Write down the number of servings you had in each food group. For Anything Goes, just write down the total number of treat calories you had. For a refresher on what counts as a serving, see page 119 in *The Best Life Diet*. And to find out how many servings of grains, fruit, and the other food groups you should have daily (and how many Anything Goes Calories you get), look at the chart on page 119 of the book. (Remember, you can also track your intake and get feedback by joining www.thebestlife.com.)

	Breakfast	Lunch	Dinner	Snack	Other	Other
Grain/Starchy Vegetables						
Fruit						
Vegetables						
Dairy (preferably nonfat or 1%)						
Protein-Rich Foods						
Fat (preferably healthy)						
Anything Goes Calories						

Are your portions becoming more reasonable?   Y   N

NOTES _____

_____

Did you stay within your Anything Goes Calories for treats?   Y   N

NOTES _____

_____

_____

_____

_____

_____

_____

_____

_____

_____

_____

_____

_____

_____

_____

_____

_____

_____

ACTIVITY LEVEL: 0   1   2   3   4   5

Aerobic minutes or steps/day _____

Did you meet your aerobic/step goal?   Y   N

NOTES _____

_____

STRENGTH TRAINING

Exercise								
Weight								
Reps								
Sets								

Did you meet your strength-training goal?   Y   N

NOTES _____

_____

Eating cutoff time: ____:____   Bedtime: ____:____

Did you cut off eating at least two hours before bedtime?   Y   N

Did you eat three meals (including a nutritious breakfast) and at least one snack?   Y   N

Did you eliminate the six problem foods from your diet?   Y   N

Did you drink at least six 8-ounce glasses of water?   Y   N

Did you take your vitamin supplements?   Y   N

                    TIME

Breakfast   ____:____   Hunger rating before eating _____   Hunger rating after eating _____

Lunch   ____:____   Hunger rating before eating _____   Hunger rating after eating _____

Dinner   ____:____   Hunger rating before eating _____   Hunger rating after eating _____

Snack   ____:____   Hunger rating before eating _____   Hunger rating after eating _____

Other meal/snack   ____:____   Hunger rating before eating _____   Hunger rating after eating _____

Other meal/snack   ____:____   Hunger rating before eating _____   Hunger rating after eating _____

Did you meet your hunger scale goals?   Y   N

NOTES _____

_____

Write down the number of servings you had in each food group. For Anything Goes, just write down the total number of treat calories you had. For a refresher on what counts as a serving, see page 119 in *The Best Life Diet*. And to find out how many servings of grains, fruit, and the other food groups you should have daily (and how many Anything Goes Calories you get), look at the chart on page 119 of the book. (Remember, you can also track your intake and get feedback by joining www.thebestlife.com.)

	Breakfast	Lunch	Dinner	Snack	Other	Other
Grain/Starchy Vegetables						
Fruit						
Vegetables						
Dairy (preferably nonfat or 1%)						
Protein-Rich Foods						
Fat (preferably healthy)						
Anything Goes Calories						

Are your portions becoming more reasonable?   Y   N

NOTES _____

_____

Did you stay within your Anything Goes Calories for treats?   Y   N

NOTES _____

_____

_____

_____

_____

_____

_____

_____

_____

_____

_____

_____

_____

_____

_____

_____

_____

Weekly Summary

Your weight: _____

Total aerobic minutes/steps for the week _____

Did you meet your aerobic/step goal?   Y   N

Did you meet your strength-training goals for the week?   Y   N

How many days did you cut off your eating at least two hours before bedtime? _____

How many days did you eat three meals and at least one snack? _____

How many days did eliminate the six problem foods? _____

How many days did you drink at least six 8-ounce glasses of water? _____

How many days did you take your vitamin supplements? _____

How many days did you meet your hunger scale goals? _____

How many days did you eat reasonable portions? _____

How many days did you stay within your Anything Goes Calories for treats? _____

How was your week overall? _____

_____

_____

_____

_____

_____

_____

_____

_____

_____

_____

_____

_____

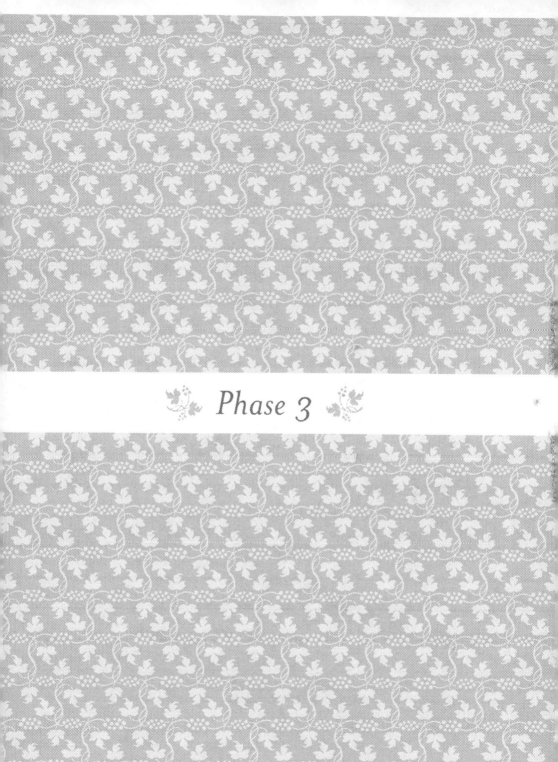

Phase 3

ACTIVITY LEVEL: 0   1   2   3   4   5

Aerobic minutes or steps/day _____

Did you meet your aerobic/step goal?   Y   N

NOTES _____

_____

STRENGTH TRAINING

Exercise								
Weight								
Reps								
Sets								

Did you meet your strength-training goal?   Y   N

NOTES _____

_____

Eating cutoff time: _____:_____   Bedtime: _____:_____

Did you cut off eating at least two hours before bedtime?   Y   N

Did you eat three meals (including a nutritious breakfast) and at least one snack?   Y   N

Did you eliminate the six problem foods from your diet?   Y   N

Did you drink at least six 8-ounce glasses of water?   Y   N

Did you take your vitamin supplements?   Y   N

                              TIME

Breakfast   _____:_____   Hunger rating before eating _____   Hunger rating after eating _____

Lunch   _____:_____   Hunger rating before eating _____   Hunger rating after eating _____

Dinner   _____:_____   Hunger rating before eating _____   Hunger rating after eating _____

Snack   _____:_____   Hunger rating before eating _____   Hunger rating after eating _____

Other meal/snack   _____:_____   Hunger rating before eating _____   Hunger rating after eating _____

Other meal/snack   _____:_____   Hunger rating before eating _____   Hunger rating after eating _____

Did you meet your hunger scale goals?   Y   N

Did you limit your intake of sodium, saturated fat, and added sugar, and eliminate trans fat?   Y   N

NOTES _____

Did you cut back on unhealthy foods and add even more wholesome foods (including whole grains, fruit,
vegetables, low-fat dairy, lean protein, and healthy fats) into your diet?   Y   N

NOTES _____

_____

Write down the number of servings you had in each food group. For Anything Goes, just write down the total number of treat calories you had. For a refresher on what counts as a serving, see page 119 in *The Best Life Diet*. And to find out how many servings of grains, fruit, and the other food groups you should have daily (and how many Anything Goes Calories you get), look at the chart on page 119 of the book. (Remember, you can also track your intake and get feedback by joining www.thebestlife.com.)

	Breakfast	Lunch	Dinner	Snack	Other	Other
Grain/Starchy Vegetables						
Fruit						
Vegetables						
Dairy (preferably nonfat or 1%)						
Protein-Rich Foods						
Fat (preferably healthy)						
Anything Goes Calories						

Are your portions becoming more reasonable?   Y   N

NOTES _____

_____

Did you stay within your Anything Goes Calories for treats?   Y   N

NOTES _____

_____

_____

_____

_____

_____

_____

_____

_____

_____

_____

_____

_____

_____

_____

_____

_____

_____

_____

ACTIVITY LEVEL: 0   1   2   3   4   5

Aerobic minutes or steps/day _____

Did you meet your aerobic/step goal?   Y   N

NOTES _____

_____

STRENGTH TRAINING

Exercise								
Weight								
Reps								
Sets								

Did you meet your strength-training goal?   Y   N

NOTES _____

_____

Eating cutoff time: ____ : ____   Bedtime: ____ : ____

Did you cut off eating at least two hours before bedtime?   Y   N

Did you eat three meals (including a nutritious breakfast) and at least one snack?   Y   N

Did you eliminate the six problem foods from your diet?   Y   N

Did you drink at least six 8-ounce glasses of water?   Y   N

Did you take your vitamin supplements?   Y   N

                         TIME

Breakfast   ____ : ____   Hunger rating before eating ____ Hunger rating after eating ____

Lunch   ____ : ____   Hunger rating before eating ____ Hunger rating after eating ____

Dinner   ____ : ____   Hunger rating before eating ____ Hunger rating after eating ____

Snack   ____ : ____   Hunger rating before eating ____ Hunger rating after eating ____

Other meal/snack ____ : ____   Hunger rating before eating ____ Hunger rating after eating ____

Other meal/snack ____ : ____   Hunger rating before eating ____ Hunger rating after eating ____

Did you meet your hunger scale goals?   Y   N

Did you limit your intake of sodium, saturated fat, and added sugar, and eliminate trans fat?   Y   N

NOTES _____

_____

Did you cut back on unhealthy foods and add even more wholesome foods (including whole grains, fruit, vegetables, low-fat dairy, lean protein, and healthy fats) into your diet?   Y   N

NOTES _____

_____

Write down the number of servings you had in each food group. For Anything Goes, just write down the total number of treat calories you had. For a refresher on what counts as a serving, see page 119 in *The Best Life Diet*. And to find out how many servings of grains, fruit, and the other food groups you should have daily (and how many Anything Goes Calories you get), look at the chart on page 119 of the book. (Remember, you can also track your intake and get feedback by joining www.thebestlife.com.)

	Breakfast	Lunch	Dinner	Snack	Other	Other
Grain/Starchy Vegetables						
Fruit						
Vegetables						
Dairy (preferably nonfat or 1%)						
Protein-Rich Foods						
Fat (preferably healthy)						
Anything Goes Calories						

Are your portions becoming more reasonable?   Y   N

NOTES _____

_____

Did you stay within your Anything Goes Calories for treats?   Y   N

NOTES _____

_____

_____

_____

_____

_____

_____

_____

_____

_____

_____

_____

_____

_____

_____

_____

_____

_____

_____

ACTIVITY LEVEL: 0   1   2   3   4   5

Aerobic minutes or steps/day _____

Did you meet your aerobic/step goal?   Y   N

NOTES _____

STRENGTH TRAINING

Exercise								
Weight								
Reps								
Sets								

Did you meet your strength-training goal?   Y   N

NOTES _____

Eating cutoff time: ___:___   Bedtime: ___:___

Did you cut off eating at least two hours before bedtime?   Y   N

Did you eat three meals (including a nutritious breakfast) and at least one snack?   Y   N

Did you eliminate the six problem foods from your diet?   Y   N

Did you drink at least six 8-ounce glasses of water?   Y   N

Did you take your vitamin supplements?   Y   N

	TIME		
Breakfast	___:___	Hunger rating before eating ___	Hunger rating after eating ___
Lunch	___:___	Hunger rating before eating ___	Hunger rating after eating ___
Dinner	___:___	Hunger rating before eating ___	Hunger rating after eating ___
Snack	___:___	Hunger rating before eating ___	Hunger rating after eating ___
Other meal/snack	___:___	Hunger rating before eating ___	Hunger rating after eating ___
Other meal/snack	___:___	Hunger rating before eating ___	Hunger rating after eating ___

Did you meet your hunger scale goals?   Y   N

Did you limit your intake of sodium, saturated fat, and added sugar, and eliminate trans fat?   Y   N

NOTES _____

Did you cut back on unhealthy foods and add even more wholesome foods (including whole grains, fruit, vegetables, low-fat dairy, lean protein, and healthy fats) into your diet?   Y   N

NOTES _____

Write down the number of servings you had in each food group. For Anything Goes, just write down the total number of treat calories you had. For a refresher on what counts as a serving, see page 119 in *The Best Life Diet*. And to find out how many servings of grains, fruit, and the other food groups you should have daily (and how many Anything Goes Calories you get), look at the chart on page 119 of the book. (Remember, you can also track your intake and get feedback by joining www.thebestlife.com.)

	Breakfast	Lunch	Dinner	Snack	Other	Other
Grain/Starchy Vegetables						
Fruit						
Vegetables						
Dairy (preferably nonfat or 1%)						
Protein-Rich Foods						
Fat (preferably healthy)						
Anything Goes Calories						

Are your portions becoming more reasonable?   Y   N

NOTES _____

_____

Did you stay within your Anything Goes Calories for treats?   Y   N

NOTES _____

_____

_____

_____

_____

_____

_____

_____

_____

_____

_____

_____

_____

_____

_____

_____

_____

ACTIVITY LEVEL: 0   1   2   3   4   5

Aerobic minutes or steps/day _____

Did you meet your aerobic/step goal?   Y   N

NOTES _____

_____

STRENGTH TRAINING

Exercise								
Weight								
Reps								
Sets								

Did you meet your strength-training goal?   Y   N

NOTES _____

_____

Eating cutoff time: ____ : ____   Bedtime: ____ : ____

Did you cut off eating at least two hours before bedtime?   Y   N

Did you eat three meals (including a nutritious breakfast) and at least one snack?   Y   N

Did you eliminate the six problem foods from your diet?   Y   N

Did you drink at least six 8-ounce glasses of water?   Y   N

Did you take your vitamin supplements?   Y   N

        TIME

Breakfast   ____ : ____   Hunger rating before eating ____   Hunger rating after eating ____

Lunch   ____ : ____   Hunger rating before eating ____   Hunger rating after eating ____

Dinner   ____ : ____   Hunger rating before eating ____   Hunger rating after eating ____

Snack   ____ : ____   Hunger rating before eating ____   Hunger rating after eating ____

Other meal/snack   ____ : ____   Hunger rating before eating ____   Hunger rating after eating ____

Other meal/snack   ____ : ____   Hunger rating before eating ____   Hunger rating after eating ____

Did you meet your hunger scale goals?   Y   N

Did you limit your intake of sodium, saturated fat, and added sugar, and eliminate trans fat?   Y   N

NOTES _____

_____

Did you cut back on unhealthy foods and add even more wholesome foods (including whole grains, fruit, vegetables, low-fat dairy, lean protein, and healthy fats) into your diet?   Y   N

NOTES _____

_____

Write down the number of servings you had in each food group. For Anything Goes, just write down the total number of treat calories you had. For a refresher on what counts as a serving, see page 119 in *The Best Life Diet*. And to find out how many servings of grains, fruit, and the other food groups you should have daily (and how many Anything Goes Calories you get), look at the chart on page 119 of the book. (Remember, you can also track your intake and get feedback by joining www.thebestlife.com.)

	Breakfast	Lunch	Dinner	Snack	Other	Other
Grain/Starchy Vegetables						
Fruit						
Vegetables						
Dairy (preferably nonfat or 1%)						
Protein-Rich Foods						
Fat (preferably healthy)						
Anything Goes Calories						

Are your portions becoming more reasonable?   Y   N

NOTES _____

_____

Did you stay within your Anything Goes Calories for treats?   Y   N

NOTES _____

_____

_____

_____

_____

_____

_____

_____

_____

_____

_____

_____

_____

_____

_____

_____

_____

_____

ACTIVITY LEVEL: 0   1   2   3   4   5

Aerobic minutes or steps/day _____

Did you meet your aerobic/step goal?   Y   N

NOTES _____

_____

STRENGTH TRAINING

Exercise								
Weight								
Reps								
Sets								

Did you meet your strength-training goal?   Y   N

NOTES _____

_____

Eating cutoff time: ____:____   Bedtime: ____:____

Did you cut off eating at least two hours before bedtime?   Y   N

Did you eat three meals (including a nutritious breakfast) and at least one snack?   Y   N

Did you eliminate the six problem foods from your diet?   Y   N

Did you drink at least six 8-ounce glasses of water?   Y   N

Did you take your vitamin supplements?   Y   N

	TIME			
Breakfast	____:____	Hunger rating before eating _____	Hunger rating after eating _____
Lunch	____:____	Hunger rating before eating _____	Hunger rating after eating _____
Dinner	____:____	Hunger rating before eating _____	Hunger rating after eating _____
Snack	____:____	Hunger rating before eating _____	Hunger rating after eating _____
Other meal/snack	____:____	Hunger rating before eating _____	Hunger rating after eating _____
Other meal/snack	____:____	Hunger rating before eating _____	Hunger rating after eating _____

Did you meet your hunger scale goals?   Y   N

Did you limit your intake of sodium, saturated fat, and added sugar, and eliminate trans fat?   Y   N

NOTES _____

_____

Did you cut back on unhealthy foods and add even more wholesome foods (including whole grains, fruit, vegetables, low-fat dairy, lean protein, and healthy fats) into your diet?   Y   N

NOTES _____

_____

Write down the number of servings you had in each food group. For Anything Goes, just write down the total number of treat calories you had. For a refresher on what counts as a serving, see page 119 in *The Best Life Diet*. And to find out how many servings of grains, fruit, and the other food groups you should have daily (and how many Anything Goes Calories you get), look at the chart on page 119 of the book. (Remember, you can also track your intake and get feedback by joining www.thebestlife.com.)

	Breakfast	Lunch	Dinner	Snack	Other	Other
Grain/Starchy Vegetables						
Fruit						
Vegetables						
Dairy (preferably nonfat or 1%)						
Protein-Rich Foods						
Fat (preferably healthy)						
Anything Goes Calories						

Are your portions becoming more reasonable?   Y   N

NOTES _____

_____

Did you stay within your Anything Goes Calories for treats?   Y   N

NOTES _____

_____

_____

_____

_____

_____

_____

_____

_____

_____

_____

_____

_____

_____

_____

_____

_____

_____

_____

ACTIVITY LEVEL: 0 1 2 3 4 5

Aerobic minutes or steps/day _____

Did you meet your aerobic/step goal?   Y   N

NOTES _____

_____

STRENGTH TRAINING

Exercise								
Weight								
Reps								
Sets								

Did you meet your strength-training goal?   Y   N

NOTES _____

_____

Eating cutoff time: ____ : ____   Bedtime: ____ : ____

Did you cut off eating at least two hours before bedtime?   Y   N

Did you eat three meals (including a nutritious breakfast) and at least one snack?   Y   N

Did you eliminate the six problem foods from your diet?   Y   N

Did you drink at least six 8-ounce glasses of water?   Y   N

Did you take your vitamin supplements?   Y   N

	TIME		
Breakfast	____ : ____	Hunger rating before eating ____	Hunger rating after eating ____
Lunch	____ : ____	Hunger rating before eating ____	Hunger rating after eating ____
Dinner	____ : ____	Hunger rating before eating ____	Hunger rating after eating ____
Snack	____ : ____	Hunger rating before eating ____	Hunger rating after eating ____
Other meal/snack	____ : ____	Hunger rating before eating ____	Hunger rating after eating ____
Other meal/snack	____ : ____	Hunger rating before eating ____	Hunger rating after eating ____

Did you meet your hunger scale goals?   Y   N

Did you limit your intake of sodium, saturated fat, and added sugar, and eliminate trans fat?   Y   N

NOTES _____

_____

Did you cut back on unhealthy foods and add even more wholesome foods (including whole grains, fruit, vegetables, low-fat dairy, lean protein, and healthy fats) into your diet?   Y   N

NOTES _____

_____

Write down the number of servings you had in each food group. For Anything Goes, just write down the total number of treat calories you had. For a refresher on what counts as a serving, see page 119 in *The Best Life Diet*. And to find out how many servings of grains, fruit, and the other food groups you should have daily (and how many Anything Goes Calories you get), look at the chart on page 119 of the book. (Remember, you can also track your intake and get feedback by joining www.thebestlife.com.)

	Breakfast	Lunch	Dinner	Snack	Other	Other
Grain/Starchy Vegetables						
Fruit						
Vegetables						
Dairy (preferably nonfat or 1%)						
Protein-Rich Foods						
Fat (preferably healthy)						
Anything Goes Calories						

Are your portions becoming more reasonable?　　　　　　　　　　　　　　Y　N

NOTES _____

_____

Did you stay within your Anything Goes Calories for treats?　　　　　Y　N

NOTES _____

_____

_____

_____

_____

_____

_____

_____

_____

_____

_____

_____

_____

_____

_____

_____

_____

ACTIVITY LEVEL: 0   1   2   3   4   5

Aerobic minutes or steps/day _____

Did you meet your aerobic/step goal?   Y   N

NOTES _____

_____

STRENGTH TRAINING

Exercise								
Weight								
Reps								
Sets								

Did you meet your strength-training goal?   Y   N

NOTES _____

_____

Eating cutoff time: ____:____   Bedtime: ____:____

Did you cut off eating at least two hours before bedtime?   Y   N

Did you eat three meals (including a nutritious breakfast) and at least one snack?   Y   N

Did you eliminate the six problem foods from your diet?   Y   N

Did you drink at least six 8-ounce glasses of water?   Y   N

Did you take your vitamin supplements?   Y   N

TIME

Breakfast   ____:____   Hunger rating before eating ____ Hunger rating after eating ____

Lunch   ____:____   Hunger rating before eating ____ Hunger rating after eating ____

Dinner   ____:____   Hunger rating before eating ____ Hunger rating after eating ____

Snack   ____:____   Hunger rating before eating ____ Hunger rating after eating ____

Other meal/snack ____:____   Hunger rating before eating ____ Hunger rating after eating ____

Other meal/snack ____:____   Hunger rating before eating ____ Hunger rating after eating ____

Did you meet your hunger scale goals?   Y   N

Did you limit your intake of sodium, saturated fat, and added sugar, and eliminate trans fat?   Y   N

NOTES _____

_____

Did you cut back on unhealthy foods and add even more wholesome foods (including whole grains, fruit, vegetables, low-fat dairy, lean protein, and healthy fats) into your diet?   Y   N

NOTES _____

_____

Write down the number of servings you had in each food group. For Anything Goes, just write down the total number of treat calories you had. For a refresher on what counts as a serving, see page 119 in *The Best Life Diet*. And to find out how many servings of grains, fruit, and the other food groups you should have daily (and how many Anything Goes Calories you get), look at the chart on page 119 of the book. (Remember, you can also track your intake and get feedback by joining www.thebestlife.com.)

	Breakfast	Lunch	Dinner	Snack	Other	Other
Grain/Starchy Vegetables						
Fruit						
Vegetables						
Dairy (preferably nonfat or 1%)						
Protein-Rich Foods						
Fat (preferably healthy)						
Anything Goes Calories						

Are your portions becoming more reasonable?   Y   N

NOTES _____

_____

Did you stay within your Anything Goes Calories for treats?   Y   N

NOTES _____

_____

_____

_____

_____

_____

_____

_____

_____

_____

_____

_____

_____

_____

_____

_____

_____

Weekly Summary

Your weight: _____

Total aerobic minutes/steps for the week   _____

Did you meet your aerobic/step goal?   Y   N

Did you meet your strength-training goals for the week?   Y   N

How many days did you cut off your eating at least two hours before bedtime?   _____

How many days did you eat three meals and at least one snack?   _____

How many days did you eliminate the six problem foods?   _____

How many days did you drink at least six 8-ounce glasses of water?   _____

How many days did you take your vitamin supplements?   _____

How many days did you meet your hunger scale goals?   _____

How many days did you limit your intake of sodium, saturated fat, and added sugar, and eliminate trans fat?   _____

How many days did you cut back on unhealthy foods and add more wholesome foods into your diet?   _____

How many days did you eat reasonable portions?   _____

How many days did you stay within your Anything Goes Calories for treats?   _____

How was your week overall?   _____

_____

_____

_____

_____

_____

_____

_____

WEEK: _____ DATE: _____ PHASE 3

ACTIVITY LEVEL: 0 1 2 3 4 5

Aerobic minutes or steps/day _____

Did you meet your aerobic/step goal?   Y N
NOTES _____
_____

STRENGTH TRAINING

Exercise								
Weight								
Reps								
Sets								

Did you meet your strength-training goal?   Y N
NOTES _____

Eating cutoff time: ____:____   Bedtime: ____:____

Did you cut off eating at least two hours before bedtime?   Y N

Did you eat three meals (including a nutritious breakfast) and at least one snack?   Y N

Did you eliminate the six problem foods from your diet?   Y N

Did you drink at least six 8-ounce glasses of water?   Y N

Did you take your vitamin supplements?   Y N

                    TIME
Breakfast   ____:____   Hunger rating before eating ____ Hunger rating after eating ____

Lunch   ____:____   Hunger rating before eating ____ Hunger rating after eating ____

Dinner   ____:____   Hunger rating before eating ____ Hunger rating after eating ____

Snack   ____:____   Hunger rating before eating ____ Hunger rating after eating ____

Other meal/snack ____:____ Hunger rating before eating ____ Hunger rating after eating ____

Other meal/snack ____:____ Hunger rating before eating ____ Hunger rating after eating ____

Did you meet your hunger scale goals?   Y N

Did you limit your intake of sodium, saturated fat, and added sugar, and eliminate trans fat?   Y N
NOTES _____

Did you cut back on unhealthy foods and add even more wholesome foods (including whole grains, fruit, vegetables, low-fat dairy, lean protein, and healthy fats) into your diet?   Y N
NOTES _____

Write down the number of servings you had in each food group. For Anything Goes, just write down the total number of treat calories you had. For a refresher on what counts as a serving, see page 119 in *The Best Life Diet*. And to find out how many servings of grains, fruit, and the other food groups you should have daily (and how many Anything Goes Calories you get), look at the chart on page 119 of the book. (Remember, you can also track your intake and get feedback by joining www.thebestlife.com.)

	Breakfast	Lunch	Dinner	Snack	Other	Other
Grain/Starchy Vegetables						
Fruit						
Vegetables						
Dairy (preferably nonfat or 1%)						
Protein-Rich Foods						
Fat (preferably healthy)						
Anything Goes Calories						

Are your portions becoming more reasonable?   Y   N

NOTES _____

_____

Did you stay within your Anything Goes Calories for treats?   Y   N

NOTES _____

_____

_____

_____

_____

_____

_____

_____

_____

_____

_____

_____

_____

_____

_____

_____

_____

_____

_____

ACTIVITY LEVEL: 0   1   2   3   4   5

Aerobic minutes or steps/day _____

Did you meet your aerobic/step goal?   Y   N

NOTES _____

_____

STRENGTH TRAINING

Exercise								
Weight								
Reps								
Sets								

Did you meet your strength-training goal?   Y   N

NOTES _____

_____

Eating cutoff time: _____:_____   Bedtime: _____:_____

Did you cut off eating at least two hours before bedtime?   Y   N

Did you eat three meals (including a nutritious breakfast) and at least one snack?   Y   N

Did you eliminate the six problem foods from your diet?   Y   N

Did you drink at least six 8-ounce glasses of water?   Y   N

Did you take your vitamin supplements?   Y   N

                              TIME

Breakfast   _____:_____   Hunger rating before eating _____   Hunger rating after eating _____

Lunch   _____:_____   Hunger rating before eating _____   Hunger rating after eating _____

Dinner   _____:_____   Hunger rating before eating _____   Hunger rating after eating _____

Snack   _____:_____   Hunger rating before eating _____   Hunger rating after eating _____

Other meal/snack   _____:_____   Hunger rating before eating _____   Hunger rating after eating _____

Other meal/snack   _____:_____   Hunger rating before eating _____   Hunger rating after eating _____

Did you meet your hunger scale goals?   Y   N

Did you limit your intake of sodium, saturated fat, and added sugar, and eliminate trans fat?   Y   N

NOTES _____

Did you cut back on unhealthy foods and add even more wholesome foods (including whole grains, fruit, vegetables, low-fat dairy, lean protein, and healthy fats) into your diet?   Y   N

NOTES _____

_____

Write down the number of servings you had in each food group. For Anything Goes, just write down the total number of treat calories you had. For a refresher on what counts as a serving, see page 119 in *The Best Life Diet*. And to find out how many servings of grains, fruit, and the other food groups you should have daily (and how many Anything Goes Calories you get), look at the chart on page 119 of the book. (Remember, you can also track your intake and get feedback by joining www.thebestlife.com.)

	Breakfast	Lunch	Dinner	Snack	Other	Other
Grain/Starchy Vegetables						
Fruit						
Vegetables						
Dairy (preferably nonfat or 1%)						
Protein-Rich Foods						
Fat (preferably healthy)						
Anything Goes Calories						

Are your portions becoming more reasonable?   Y   N

NOTES_____

_____

Did you stay within your Anything Goes Calories for treats?   Y   N

NOTES_____

_____

_____

_____

_____

_____

_____

_____

_____

_____

_____

_____

_____

_____

_____

_____

_____

_____

_____

ACTIVITY LEVEL: 0   1   2   3   4   5

Aerobic minutes or steps/day _____

Did you meet your aerobic/step goal?   Y   N

NOTES _____

_____

STRENGTH TRAINING

Exercise								
Weight								
Reps								
Sets								

Did you meet your strength-training goal?   Y   N

NOTES _____

_____

Eating cutoff time: ____:____   Bedtime: ____:____

Did you cut off eating at least two hours before bedtime?   Y   N

Did you eat three meals (including a nutritious breakfast) and at least one snack?   Y   N

Did you eliminate the six problem foods from your diet?   Y   N

Did you drink at least six 8-ounce glasses of water?   Y   N

Did you take your vitamin supplements?   Y   N

                  TIME

Breakfast   ____:____   Hunger rating before eating _____   Hunger rating after eating _____

Lunch   ____:____   Hunger rating before eating _____   Hunger rating after eating _____

Dinner   ____:____   Hunger rating before eating _____   Hunger rating after eating _____

Snack   ____:____   Hunger rating before eating _____   Hunger rating after eating _____

Other meal/snack ____:____   Hunger rating before eating _____   Hunger rating after eating _____

Other meal/snack ____:____   Hunger rating before eating _____   Hunger rating after eating _____

Did you meet your hunger scale goals?   Y   N

Did you limit your intake of sodium, saturated fat, and added sugar, and eliminate trans fat?   Y   N

NOTES _____

_____

Did you cut back on unhealthy foods and add even more wholesome foods (including whole grains, fruit, vegetables, low-fat dairy, lean protein, and healthy fats) into your diet?   Y   N

NOTES _____

_____

Write down the number of servings you had in each food group. For Anything Goes, just write down the total number of treat calories you had. For a refresher on what counts as a serving, see page 119 in *The Best Life Diet*. And to find out how many servings of grains, fruit, and the other food groups you should have daily (and how many Anything Goes Calories you get), look at the chart on page 119 of the book. (Remember, you can also track your intake and get feedback by joining www.thebestlife.com.)

	Breakfast	Lunch	Dinner	Snack	Other	Other
Grain/Starchy Vegetables						
Fruit						
Vegetables						
Dairy (preferably nonfat or 1%)						
Protein-Rich Foods						
Fat (preferably healthy)						
Anything Goes Calories						

Are your portions becoming more reasonable?   Y   N

NOTES _____

_____

Did you stay within your Anything Goes Calories for treats?   Y   N

NOTES _____

_____

_____

_____

_____

_____

_____

_____

_____

_____

_____

_____

_____

_____

_____

_____

_____

_____

WEEK: **DATE:** PHASE 3

Aerobic minutes or steps/day _____

Did you meet your aerobic/step goal?   Y   N

NOTES _____

_____

STRENGTH TRAINING

Exercise							
Weight							
Reps							
Sets							

Did you meet your strength-training goal?   Y   N

NOTES _____

_____

Eating cutoff time: ____:____   Bedtime: ____:____

Did you cut off eating at least two hours before bedtime?   Y   N

Did you eat three meals (including a nutritious breakfast) and at least one snack?   Y   N

Did you eliminate the six problem foods from your diet?   Y   N

Did you drink at least six 8-ounce glasses of water?   Y   N

Did you take your vitamin supplements?   Y   N

TIME

Breakfast   ____:____   Hunger rating before eating ____ Hunger rating after eating ____

Lunch   ____:____   Hunger rating before eating ____ Hunger rating after eating ____

Dinner   ____:____   Hunger rating before eating ____ Hunger rating after eating ____

Snack   ____:____   Hunger rating before eating ____ Hunger rating after eating ____

Other meal/snack   ____:____   Hunger rating before eating ____ Hunger rating after eating ____

Other meal/snack   ____:____   Hunger rating before eating ____ Hunger rating after eating ____

Did you meet your hunger scale goals?   Y   N

Did you limit your intake of sodium, saturated fat, and added sugar, and eliminate trans fat? Y   N

NOTES _____

_____

Did you cut back on unhealthy foods and add even more wholesome foods (including whole grains, fruit, vegetables, low-fat dairy, lean protein, and healthy fats) into your diet?   Y   N

NOTES _____

_____

Write down the number of servings you had in each food group. For Anything Goes, just write down the total number of treat calories you had. For a refresher on what counts as a serving, see page 119 in *The Best Life Diet*. And to find out how many servings of grains, fruit, and the other food groups you should have daily (and how many Anything Goes Calories you get), look at the chart on page 119 of the book. (Remember, you can also track your intake and get feedback by joining www.thebestlife.com.)

	Breakfast	Lunch	Dinner	Snack	Other	Other
Grain/Starchy Vegetables						
Fruit						
Vegetables						
Dairy (preferably nonfat or 1%)						
Protein-Rich Foods						
Fat (preferably healthy)						
Anything Goes Calories						

Are your portions becoming more reasonable?   Y   N

NOTES _____

_____

Did you stay within your Anything Goes Calories for treats?   Y   N

NOTES _____

_____

_____

_____

_____

_____

_____

_____

_____

_____

_____

_____

_____

_____

_____

_____

_____

_____

_____

ACTIVITY LEVEL: 0   1   2   3   4   5

Aerobic minutes or steps/day _____

Did you meet your aerobic/step goal?   Y   N

NOTES _____

_____

STRENGTH TRAINING

Exercise								
Weight								
Reps								
Sets								

Did you meet your strength-training goal?   Y   N

NOTES _____

Eating cutoff time: ____:____   Bedtime: ____:____

Did you cut off eating at least two hours before bedtime?   Y   N

Did you eat three meals (including a nutritious breakfast) and at least one snack?   Y   N

Did you eliminate the six problem foods from your diet?   Y   N

Did you drink at least six 8-ounce glasses of water?   Y   N

Did you take your vitamin supplements?   Y   N

	TIME		
Breakfast	____:____	Hunger rating before eating ____	Hunger rating after eating ____
Lunch	____:____	Hunger rating before eating ____	Hunger rating after eating ____
Dinner	____:____	Hunger rating before eating ____	Hunger rating after eating ____
Snack	____:____	Hunger rating before eating ____	Hunger rating after eating ____
Other meal/snack	____:____	Hunger rating before eating ____	Hunger rating after eating ____
Other meal/snack	____:____	Hunger rating before eating ____	Hunger rating after eating ____

Did you meet your hunger scale goals?   Y   N

Did you limit your intake of sodium, saturated fat, and added sugar, and eliminate trans fat?   Y   N

NOTES _____

Did you cut back on unhealthy foods and add even more wholesome foods (including whole grains, fruit, vegetables, low-fat dairy, lean protein, and healthy fats) into your diet?   Y   N

NOTES _____

Write down the number of servings you had in each food group. For Anything Goes, just write down the total number of treat calories you had. For a refresher on what counts as a serving, see page 119 in *The Best Life Diet*. And to find out how many servings of grains, fruit, and the other food groups you should have daily (and how many Anything Goes Calories you get), look at the chart on page 119 of the book. (Remember, you can also track your intake and get feedback by joining www.thebestlife.com.)

	Breakfast	Lunch	Dinner	Snack	Other	Other
Grain/Starchy Vegetables						
Fruit						
Vegetables						
Dairy (preferably nonfat or 1%)						
Protein-Rich Foods						
Fat (preferably healthy)						
Anything Goes Calories						

Are your portions becoming more reasonable?   Y   N

NOTES _____

_____

Did you stay within your Anything Goes Calories for treats?   Y   N

NOTES _____

_____

_____

_____

_____

_____

_____

_____

_____

_____

_____

_____

_____

_____

_____

_____

_____

_____

ACTIVITY LEVEL: 0 1 2 3 4 5

Aerobic minutes or steps/day _____

Did you meet your aerobic/step goal?   Y   N

NOTES _____

_____

STRENGTH TRAINING

Exercise								
Weight								
Reps								
Sets								

Did you meet your strength-training goal?   Y   N

NOTES _____

Eating cutoff time: _____ : _____   Bedtime: _____ : _____

Did you cut off eating at least two hours before bedtime?   Y   N

Did you eat three meals (including a nutritious breakfast) and at least one snack?   Y   N

Did you eliminate the six problem foods from your diet?   Y   N

Did you drink at least six 8-ounce glasses of water?   Y   N

Did you take your vitamin supplements?   Y   N

               TIME

Breakfast   _____ : _____   Hunger rating before eating _____   Hunger rating after eating _____

Lunch   _____ : _____   Hunger rating before eating _____   Hunger rating after eating _____

Dinner   _____ : _____   Hunger rating before eating _____   Hunger rating after eating _____

Snack   _____ : _____   Hunger rating before eating _____   Hunger rating after eating _____

Other meal/snack _____ : _____   Hunger rating before eating _____   Hunger rating after eating _____

Other meal/snack _____ : _____   Hunger rating before eating _____   Hunger rating after eating _____

Did you meet your hunger scale goals?   Y   N

Did you limit your intake of sodium, saturated fat, and added sugar, and eliminate trans fat?   Y   N

NOTES _____

Did you cut back on unhealthy foods and add even more wholesome foods (including whole grains, fruit, vegetables, low-fat dairy, lean protein, and healthy fats) into your diet?   Y   N

NOTES _____

Write down the number of servings you had in each food group. For Anything Goes, just write down the total number of treat calories you had. For a refresher on what counts as a serving, see page 119 in *The Best Life Diet*. And to find out how many servings of grains, fruit, and the other food groups you should have daily (and how many Anything Goes Calories you get), look at the chart on page 119 of the book. (Remember, you can also track your intake and get feedback by joining www.thebestlife.com.)

	Breakfast	Lunch	Dinner	Snack	Other	Other
Grain/Starchy Vegetables						
Fruit						
Vegetables						
Dairy (preferably nonfat or 1%)						
Protein-Rich Foods						
Fat (preferably healthy)						
Anything Goes Calories						

Are your portions becoming more reasonable?　　　　　　　　　　　　　　Y　N

NOTES _____

_____

Did you stay within your Anything Goes Calories for treats?　　　　　　　Y　N

NOTES _____

_____

_____

_____

_____

_____

_____

_____

_____

_____

_____

_____

_____

_____

_____

_____

_____

ACTIVITY LEVEL: 0   1   2   3   4   5

Aerobic minutes or steps/day _____

Did you meet your aerobic/step goal?   Y   N

NOTES _____

_____

STRENGTH TRAINING

Exercise							
Weight							
Reps							
Sets							

Did you meet your strength-training goal?   Y   N

NOTES _____

Eating cutoff time: ____:____   Bedtime: ____:____

Did you cut off eating at least two hours before bedtime?   Y   N

Did you eat three meals (including a nutritious breakfast) and at least one snack? Y   N

Did you eliminate the six problem foods from your diet?   Y   N

Did you drink at least six 8-ounce glasses of water?   Y   N

Did you take your vitamin supplements?   Y   N

              TIME

Breakfast   ____:____   Hunger rating before eating ____   Hunger rating after eating ____

Lunch   ____:____   Hunger rating before eating ____   Hunger rating after eating ____

Dinner   ____:____   Hunger rating before eating ____   Hunger rating after eating ____

Snack   ____:____   Hunger rating before eating ____   Hunger rating after eating ____

Other meal/snack ____:____   Hunger rating before eating ____   Hunger rating after eating ____

Other meal/snack ____:____   Hunger rating before eating ____   Hunger rating after eating ____

Did you meet your hunger scale goals?   Y   N

Did you limit your intake of sodium, saturated fat, and added sugar, and eliminate trans fat?   Y   N

NOTES _____

Did you cut back on unhealthy foods and add even more wholesome foods (including whole grains, fruit, vegetables, low-fat dairy, lean protein, and healthy fats) into your diet?   Y   N

NOTES _____

Write down the number of servings you had in each food group. For Anything Goes, just write down the total number of treat calories you had. For a refresher on what counts as a serving, see page 119 in *The Best Life Diet*. And to find out how many servings of grains, fruit, and the other food groups you should have daily (and how many Anything Goes Calories you get), look at the chart on page 119 of the book. (Remember, you can also track your intake and get feedback by joining www.thebestlife.com.)

	Breakfast	Lunch	Dinner	Snack	Other	Other
Grain/Starchy Vegetables						
Fruit						
Vegetables						
Dairy (preferably nonfat or 1%)						
Protein-Rich Foods						
Fat (preferably healthy)						
Anything Goes Calories						

Are your portions becoming more reasonable?   Y   N
NOTES _____
_____

Did you stay within your Anything Goes Calories for treats?   Y   N
NOTES _____
_____
_____
_____
_____
_____
_____
_____
_____
_____
_____
_____
_____
_____
_____
_____
_____

Weekly Summary

Your weight: _____

Total aerobic minutes/steps for the week   _____

Did you meet your aerobic/step goal?   Y N

Did you meet your strength-training goals for the week?   Y N

How many days did you cut off your eating at least two hours before bedtime? _____

How many days did you eat three meals and at least one snack? _____

How many days did you eliminate the six problem foods? _____

How many days did you drink at least six 8-ounce glasses of water? _____

How many days did you take your vitamin supplements? _____

How many days did you meet your hunger scale goals? _____

How many days did you limit your intake of sodium, saturated fat and added sugar and eliminate trans fat? _____

How many days did you cut back on unhealthy foods and add more wholesome foods into your diet? _____

How many days did you eat reasonable portions? _____

How many days did you stay within your Anything Goes Calories for treats? _____

How was your week overall? _____

_____

_____

_____

_____

_____

_____

_____

_____

_____

ACTIVITY LEVEL: 0   1   2   3   4   5

Aerobic minutes or steps/day _____

Did you meet your aerobic/step goal?   Y   N

NOTES _____

STRENGTH TRAINING

Exercise								
Weight								
Reps								
Sets								

Did you meet your strength-training goal?   Y   N

NOTES _____

Eating cutoff time: _____ : _____   Bedtime: _____ : _____

Did you cut off eating at least two hours before bedtime?   Y   N

Did you eat three meals (including a nutritious breakfast) and at least one snack?   Y   N

Did you eliminate the six problem foods from your diet?   Y   N

Did you drink at least six 8-ounce glasses of water?   Y   N

Did you take your vitamin supplements?   Y   N

                     TIME

Breakfast   _____ : _____   Hunger rating before eating _____   Hunger rating after eating _____

Lunch   _____ : _____   Hunger rating before eating _____   Hunger rating after eating _____

Dinner   _____ : _____   Hunger rating before eating _____   Hunger rating after eating _____

Snack   _____ : _____   Hunger rating before eating _____   Hunger rating after eating _____

Other meal/snack _____ : _____   Hunger rating before eating _____   Hunger rating after eating _____

Other meal/snack _____ : _____   Hunger rating before eating _____   Hunger rating after eating _____

Did you meet your hunger scale goals?   Y   N

Did you limit your intake of sodium, saturated fat, and added sugar, and eliminate trans fat?   Y   N

NOTES _____

Did you cut back on unhealthy foods and add even more wholesome foods (including whole grains, fruit, vegetables, low-fat dairy, lean protein, and healthy fats) into your diet?   Y   N

NOTES _____

Write down the number of servings you had in each food group. For Anything Goes, just write down the total number of treat calories you had. For a refresher on what counts as a serving, see page 119 in *The Best Life Diet*. And to find out how many servings of grains, fruit, and the other food groups you should have daily (and how many Anything Goes Calories you get), look at the chart on page 119 of the book. (Remember, you can also track your intake and get feedback by joining www.thebestlife.com.)

	Breakfast	Lunch	Dinner	Snack	Other	Other
Grain/Starchy Vegetables						
Fruit						
Vegetables						
Dairy (preferably nonfat or 1%)						
Protein-Rich Foods						
Fat (preferably healthy)						
Anything Goes Calories						

Are your portions becoming more reasonable?   Y   N

NOTES _____

_____

Did you stay within your Anything Goes Calories for treats?   Y   N

NOTES _____

_____

_____

_____

_____

_____

_____

_____

_____

_____

_____

_____

_____

_____

_____

_____

_____

_____

ACTIVITY LEVEL: 0   1   2   3   4   5

Aerobic minutes or steps/day _____

Did you meet your aerobic/step goal?   Y   N

NOTES _____

_____

STRENGTH TRAINING

Exercise								
Weight								
Reps								
Sets								

Did you meet your strength-training goal?   Y   N

NOTES _____

_____

Eating cutoff time: ____ : ____   Bedtime: ____ : ____

Did you cut off eating at least two hours before bedtime?   Y   N

Did you eat three meals (including a nutritious breakfast) and at least one snack?   Y   N

Did you eliminate the six problem foods from your diet?   Y   N

Did you drink at least six 8-ounce glasses of water?   Y   N

Did you take your vitamin supplements?   Y   N

                        TIME

Breakfast   ____ : ____   Hunger rating before eating _____ Hunger rating after eating _____

Lunch   ____ : ____   Hunger rating before eating _____ Hunger rating after eating _____

Dinner   ____ : ____   Hunger rating before eating _____ Hunger rating after eating _____

Snack   ____ : ____   Hunger rating before eating _____ Hunger rating after eating _____

Other meal/snack ____ : ____   Hunger rating before eating _____ Hunger rating after eating _____

Other meal/snack ____ : ____   Hunger rating before eating _____ Hunger rating after eating _____

Did you meet your hunger scale goals?   Y   N

Did you limit your intake of sodium, saturated fat, and added sugar, and eliminate trans fat?   Y   N

NOTES _____

_____

Did you cut back on unhealthy foods and add even more wholesome foods (including whole grains, fruit, vegetables, low-fat dairy, lean protein, and healthy fats) into your diet?   Y   N

NOTES _____

_____

Write down the number of servings you had in each food group. For Anything Goes, just write down the total number of treat calories you had. For a refresher on what counts as a serving, see page 119 in *The Best Life Diet*. And to find out how many servings of grains, fruit, and the other food groups you should have daily (and how many Anything Goes Calories you get), look at the chart on page 119 of the book. (Remember, you can also track your intake and get feedback by joining www.thebestlife.com.)

	Breakfast	Lunch	Dinner	Snack	Other	Other
Grain/Starchy Vegetables						
Fruit						
Vegetables						
Dairy (preferably nonfat or 1%)						
Protein-Rich Foods						
Fat (preferably healthy)						
Anything Goes Calories						

Are your portions becoming more reasonable?   Y   N

NOTES _____

_____

Did you stay within your Anything Goes Calories for treats?   Y   N

NOTES _____

_____

_____

_____

_____

_____

_____

_____

_____

_____

_____

_____

_____

_____

_____

_____

_____

_____

ACTIVITY LEVEL: 0   1   2   3   4   5

Aerobic minutes or steps/day _____

Did you meet your aerobic/step goal?   Y   N

NOTES _____

_____

STRENGTH TRAINING

Exercise								
Weight								
Reps								
Sets								

Did you meet your strength-training goal?   Y   N

NOTES _____

_____

Eating cutoff time: ____:____   Bedtime: ____:____

Did you cut off eating at least two hours before bedtime?   Y   N

Did you eat three meals (including a nutritious breakfast) and at least one snack?   Y   N

Did you eliminate the six problem foods from your diet?   Y   N

Did you drink at least six 8-ounce glasses of water?   Y   N

Did you take your vitamin supplements?   Y   N

TIME

Breakfast   ____:____   Hunger rating before eating ____   Hunger rating after eating ____

Lunch   ____:____   Hunger rating before eating ____   Hunger rating after eating ____

Dinner   ____:____   Hunger rating before eating ____   Hunger rating after eating ____

Snack   ____:____   Hunger rating before eating ____   Hunger rating after eating ____

Other meal/snack ____:____   Hunger rating before eating ____   Hunger rating after eating ____

Other meal/snack ____:____   Hunger rating before eating ____   Hunger rating after eating ____

Did you meet your hunger scale goals?   Y   N

Did you limit your intake of sodium, saturated fat, and added sugar, and eliminate trans fat?   Y   N

NOTES _____

_____

Did you cut back on unhealthy foods and add even more wholesome foods (including whole grains, fruit, vegetables, low-fat dairy, lean protein, and healthy fats) into your diet?   Y   N

NOTES _____

_____

Write down the number of servings you had in each food group. For Anything Goes, just write down the total number of treat calories you had. For a refresher on what counts as a serving, see page 119 in *The Best Life Diet*. And to find out how many servings of grains, fruit, and the other food groups you should have daily (and how many Anything Goes Calories you get), look at the chart on page 119 of the book. (Remember, you can also track your intake and get feedback by joining www.thebestlife.com.)

	Breakfast	Lunch	Dinner	Snack	Other	Other
Grain/Starchy Vegetables						
Fruit						
Vegetables						
Dairy (preferably nonfat or 1%)						
Protein-Rich Foods						
Fat (preferably healthy)						
Anything Goes Calories						

Are your portions becoming more reasonable?   Y   N

NOTES _____

_____

Did you stay within your Anything Goes Calories for treats?   Y   N

NOTES _____

_____

_____

_____

_____

_____

_____

_____

_____

_____

_____

_____

_____

_____

_____

_____

_____

ACTIVITY LEVEL: 0 1 2 3 4 5

Aerobic minutes or steps/day _____

Did you meet your aerobic/step goal?   Y N

NOTES _____

_____

STRENGTH TRAINING

Exercise								
Weight								
Reps								
Sets								

Did you meet your strength-training goal?   Y N

NOTES _____

_____

Eating cutoff time: _____:_____   Bedtime: _____:_____

Did you cut off eating at least two hours before bedtime?   Y N

Did you eat three meals (including a nutritious breakfast) and at least one snack?   Y N

Did you eliminate the six problem foods from your diet?   Y N

Did you drink at least six 8-ounce glasses of water?   Y N

Did you take your vitamin supplements?   Y N

                        TIME

Breakfast   _____:_____   Hunger rating before eating _____ Hunger rating after eating _____

Lunch   _____:_____   Hunger rating before eating _____ Hunger rating after eating _____

Dinner   _____:_____   Hunger rating before eating _____ Hunger rating after eating _____

Snack   _____:_____   Hunger rating before eating _____ Hunger rating after eating _____

Other meal/snack _____:_____   Hunger rating before eating _____ Hunger rating after eating _____

Other meal/snack _____:_____   Hunger rating before eating _____ Hunger rating after eating _____

Did you meet your hunger scale goals?   Y N

Did you limit your intake of sodium, saturated fat, and added sugar, and eliminate trans fat?   Y N

NOTES _____

_____

Did you cut back on unhealthy foods and add even more wholesome foods (including whole grains, fruit, vegetables, low-fat dairy, lean protein, and healthy fats) into your diet?   Y N

NOTES _____

_____

Write down the number of servings you had in each food group. For Anything Goes, just write down the total number of treat calories you had. For a refresher on what counts as a serving, see page 119 in *The Best Life Diet*. And to find out how many servings of grains, fruit, and the other food groups you should have daily (and how many Anything Goes Calories you get), look at the chart on page 119 of the book. (Remember, you can also track your intake and get feedback by joining www.thebestlife.com.)

	Breakfast	Lunch	Dinner	Snack	Other	Other
Grain/Starchy Vegetables						
Fruit						
Vegetables						
Dairy (preferably nonfat or 1%)						
Protein-Rich Foods						
Fat (preferably healthy)						
Anything Goes Calories						

Are your portions becoming more reasonable?   Y   N

NOTES _____

_____

Did you stay within your Anything Goes Calories for treats?   Y   N

NOTES _____

_____

_____

_____

_____

_____

_____

_____

_____

_____

_____

_____

_____

_____

_____

_____

_____

_____

ACTIVITY LEVEL: 0 1 2 3 4 5

Aerobic minutes or steps/day _____

Did you meet your aerobic/step goal? Y N

NOTES _____

_____

STRENGTH TRAINING

Exercise								
Weight								
Reps								
Sets								

Did you meet your strength-training goal? Y N

NOTES _____

_____

Eating cutoff time: ____ : ____   Bedtime: ____ : ____

Did you cut off eating at least two hours before bedtime? Y N

Did you eat three meals (including a nutritious breakfast) and at least one snack? Y N

Did you eliminate the six problem foods from your diet? Y N

Did you drink at least six 8-ounce glasses of water? Y N

Did you take your vitamin supplements? Y N

	TIME		
Breakfast	____ : ____	Hunger rating before eating ____	Hunger rating after eating ____
Lunch	____ : ____	Hunger rating before eating ____	Hunger rating after eating ____
Dinner	____ : ____	Hunger rating before eating ____	Hunger rating after eating ____
Snack	____ : ____	Hunger rating before eating ____	Hunger rating after eating ____
Other meal/snack	____ : ____	Hunger rating before eating ____	Hunger rating after eating ____
Other meal/snack	____ : ____	Hunger rating before eating ____	Hunger rating after eating ____

Did you meet your hunger scale goals? Y N

Did you limit your intake of sodium, saturated fat, and added sugar, and eliminate trans fat? Y N

NOTES _____

_____

Did you cut back on unhealthy foods and add even more wholesome foods (including whole grains, fruit, vegetables, low-fat dairy, lean protein, and healthy fats) into your diet? Y N

NOTES _____

_____

Write down the number of servings you had in each food group. For Anything Goes, just write down the total number of treat calories you had. For a refresher on what counts as a serving, see page 119 in *The Best Life Diet*. And to find out how many servings of grains, fruit, and the other food groups you should have daily (and how many Anything Goes Calories you get), look at the chart on page 119 of the book. (Remember, you can also track your intake and get feedback by joining www.thebestlife.com.)

	Breakfast	Lunch	Dinner	Snack	Other	Other
Grain/Starchy Vegetables						
Fruit						
Vegetables						
Dairy (preferably nonfat or 1%)						
Protein-Rich Foods						
Fat (preferably healthy)						
Anything Goes Calories						

Are your portions becoming more reasonable?   Y   N
NOTES _____
_____

Did you stay within your Anything Goes Calories for treats?   Y   N
NOTES _____
_____
_____
_____
_____
_____
_____
_____
_____
_____
_____
_____
_____
_____
_____
_____
_____
_____

ACTIVITY LEVEL: 0 1 2 3 4 5

Aerobic minutes or steps/day _____

Did you meet your aerobic/step goal? Y N

NOTES _____

_____

STRENGTH TRAINING

Exercise							
Weight							
Reps							
Sets							

Did you meet your strength-training goal? Y N

NOTES _____

Eating cutoff time: ____:____ Bedtime: ____:____

Did you cut off eating at least two hours before bedtime? Y N

Did you eat three meals (including a nutritious breakfast) and at least one snack? Y N

Did you eliminate the six problem foods from your diet? Y N

Did you drink at least six 8-ounce glasses of water? Y N

Did you take your vitamin supplements? Y N

TIME

Breakfast ____:____ Hunger rating before eating _____ Hunger rating after eating _____

Lunch ____:____ Hunger rating before eating _____ Hunger rating after eating _____

Dinner ____:____ Hunger rating before eating _____ Hunger rating after eating _____

Snack ____:____ Hunger rating before eating _____ Hunger rating after eating _____

Other meal/snack ____:____ Hunger rating before eating _____ Hunger rating after eating _____

Other meal/snack ____:____ Hunger rating before eating _____ Hunger rating after eating _____

Did you meet your hunger scale goals? Y N

Did you limit your intake of sodium, saturated fat, and added sugar, and eliminate trans fat? Y N

NOTES _____

Did you cut back on unhealthy foods and add even more wholesome foods (including whole grains, fruit, vegetables, low-fat dairy, lean protein, and healthy fats) into your diet? Y N

NOTES _____

Write down the number of servings you had in each food group. For Anything Goes, just write down the total number of treat calories you had. For a refresher on what counts as a serving, see page 119 in *The Best Life Diet*. And to find out how many servings of grains, fruit, and the other food groups you should have daily (and how many Anything Goes Calories you get), look at the chart on page 119 of the book. (Remember, you can also track your intake and get feedback by joining www.thebestlife.com.)

	Breakfast	Lunch	Dinner	Snack	Other	Other
Grain/Starchy Vegetables						
Fruit						
Vegetables						
Dairy (preferably nonfat or 1%)						
Protein-Rich Foods						
Fat (preferably healthy)						
Anything Goes Calories						

Are your portions becoming more reasonable?   Y   N

NOTES _____

_____

Did you stay within your Anything Goes Calories for treats?   Y   N

NOTES _____

_____

_____

_____

_____

_____

_____

_____

_____

_____

_____

_____

_____

_____

_____

_____

_____

_____

_____

ACTIVITY LEVEL: 0 1 2 3 4 5

Aerobic minutes or steps/day _____

Did you meet your aerobic/step goal?   Y N

NOTES _____

_____

STRENGTH TRAINING

Exercise								
Weight								
Reps								
Sets								

Did you meet your strength-training goal?   Y N

NOTES _____

Eating cutoff time: ___:___   Bedtime: ___:___

Did you cut off eating at least two hours before bedtime?   Y N

Did you eat three meals (including a nutritious breakfast) and at least one snack?   Y N

Did you eliminate the six problem foods from your diet?   Y N

Did you drink at least six 8-ounce glasses of water?   Y N

Did you take your vitamin supplements?   Y N

	TIME		
Breakfast	___:___	Hunger rating before eating ___	Hunger rating after eating ___
Lunch	___:___	Hunger rating before eating ___	Hunger rating after eating ___
Dinner	___:___	Hunger rating before eating ___	Hunger rating after eating ___
Snack	___:___	Hunger rating before eating ___	Hunger rating after eating ___
Other meal/snack	___:___	Hunger rating before eating ___	Hunger rating after eating ___
Other meal/snack	___:___	Hunger rating before eating ___	Hunger rating after eating ___

Did you meet your hunger scale goals?   Y N

Did you limit your intake of sodium, saturated fat, and added sugar, and eliminate trans fat?   Y N

NOTES _____

_____

Did you cut back on unhealthy foods and add even more wholesome foods (including whole grains, fruit, vegetables, low-fat dairy, lean protein, and healthy fats) into your diet?   Y N

NOTES _____

Write down the number of servings you had in each food group. For Anything Goes, just write down the total number of treat calories you had. For a refresher on what counts as a serving, see page 119 in *The Best Life Diet*. And to find out how many servings of grains, fruit, and the other food groups you should have daily (and how many Anything Goes Calories you get), look at the chart on page 119 of the book. (Remember, you can also track your intake and get feedback by joining www.thebestlife.com.)

	Breakfast	Lunch	Dinner	Snack	Other	Other
Grain/Starchy Vegetables						
Fruit						
Vegetables						
Dairy (preferably nonfat or 1%)						
Protein-Rich Foods						
Fat (preferably healthy)						
Anything Goes Calories						

Are your portions becoming more reasonable?   Y   N

NOTES _____

_____

Did you stay within your Anything Goes Calories for treats?   Y   N

NOTES _____

_____

_____

_____

_____

_____

_____

_____

_____

_____

_____

_____

_____

_____

_____

_____

_____

_____

Weekly Summary

WEEK: _____   PHASE 3

Your weight: _____

Total aerobic minutes/steps for the week _____

Did you meet your aerobic/step goal?   Y   N

Did you meet your strength-training goals for the week?   Y   N

How many days did you cut off your eating at least two hours before bedtime? _____

How many days did you eat three meals and at least one snack? _____

How many days did you eliminate the six problem foods? _____

How many days did you drink at least six 8-ounce glasses of water? _____

How many days did you take your vitamin supplements? _____

How many days did you meet your hunger scale goals? _____

How many days did you limit your intake of sodium, saturated fat and added
sugar and eliminate trans fat? _____

How many days did you cut back on unhealthy foods and add more wholesome
foods into your diet? _____

How many days did you eat reasonable portions? _____

How many days did you stay within your Anything Goes Calories for treats? _____

How was your week overall? _____

_____

_____

_____

_____

_____

_____

_____

_____

_____

ACTIVITY LEVEL: 0   1   2   3   4   5

Aerobic minutes or steps/day _____

Did you meet your aerobic/step goal?   Y   N

NOTES _____

_____

STRENGTH TRAINING

Exercise								
Weight								
Reps								
Sets								

Did you meet your strength-training goal?   Y   N

NOTES _____

_____

Eating cutoff time: ____:____   Bedtime: ____:____

Did you cut off eating at least two hours before bedtime?   Y   N

Did you eat three meals (including a nutritious breakfast) and at least one snack?   Y   N

Did you eliminate the six problem foods from your diet?   Y   N

Did you drink at least six 8-ounce glasses of water?   Y   N

Did you take your vitamin supplements?   Y   N

                    TIME

Breakfast   ____:____   Hunger rating before eating _____ Hunger rating after eating _____

Lunch   ____:____   Hunger rating before eating _____ Hunger rating after eating _____

Dinner   ____:____   Hunger rating before eating _____ Hunger rating after eating _____

Snack   ____:____   Hunger rating before eating _____ Hunger rating after eating _____

Other meal/snack ____:____   Hunger rating before eating _____ Hunger rating after eating _____

Other meal/snack ____:____   Hunger rating before eating _____ Hunger rating after eating _____

Did you meet your hunger scale goals?   Y   N

Did you limit your intake of sodium, saturated fat, and added sugar, and eliminate trans fat?   Y   N

NOTES _____

_____

Did you cut back on unhealthy foods and add even more wholesome foods (including whole grains, fruit, vegetables, low-fat dairy, lean protein, and healthy fats) into your diet?   Y   N

NOTES _____

_____

Write down the number of servings you had in each food group. For Anything Goes, just write down the total number of treat calories you had. For a refresher on what counts as a serving, see page 119 in *The Best Life Diet*. And to find out how many servings of grains, fruit, and the other food groups you should have daily (and how many Anything Goes Calories you get), look at the chart on page 119 of the book. (Remember, you can also track your intake and get feedback by joining www.thebestlife.com.)

	Breakfast	Lunch	Dinner	Snack	Other	Other
Grain/Starchy Vegetables						
Fruit						
Vegetables						
Dairy (preferably nonfat or 1%)						
Protein-Rich Foods						
Fat (preferably healthy)						
Anything Goes Calories						

Are your portions becoming more reasonable?   Y   N

NOTES _____

_____

Did you stay within your Anything Goes Calories for treats?   Y   N

NOTES _____

_____

_____

_____

_____

_____

_____

_____

_____

_____

_____

_____

_____

_____

_____

_____

_____

_____

ACTIVITY LEVEL: 0   1   2   3   4   5

Aerobic minutes or steps/day _____

Did you meet your aerobic/step goal?   Y   N

NOTES _____

_____

STRENGTH TRAINING

Exercise							
Weight							
Reps							
Sets							

Did you meet your strength-training goal?   Y   N

NOTES _____

_____

Eating cutoff time: ____ : ____   Bedtime: ____ : ____

Did you cut off eating at least two hours before bedtime?   Y   N

Did you eat three meals (including a nutritious breakfast) and at least one snack?   Y   N

Did you eliminate the six problem foods from your diet?   Y   N

Did you drink at least six 8-ounce glasses of water?   Y   N

Did you take your vitamin supplements?   Y   N

                          TIME

Breakfast   ____ : ____   Hunger rating before eating ____   Hunger rating after eating ____

Lunch   ____ : ____   Hunger rating before eating ____   Hunger rating after eating ____

Dinner   ____ : ____   Hunger rating before eating ____   Hunger rating after eating ____

Snack   ____ : ____   Hunger rating before eating ____   Hunger rating after eating ____

Other meal/snack ____ : ____   Hunger rating before eating ____   Hunger rating after eating ____

Other meal/snack ____ : ____   Hunger rating before eating ____   Hunger rating after eating ____

Did you meet your hunger scale goals?   Y   N

Did you limit your intake of sodium, saturated fat, and added sugar, and eliminate trans fat?   Y   N

NOTES _____

_____

Did you cut back on unhealthy foods and add even more wholesome foods (including whole grains, fruit, vegetables, low-fat dairy, lean protein, and healthy fats) into your diet?   Y   N

NOTES _____

_____

Write down the number of servings you had in each food group. For Anything Goes, just write down the total number of treat calories you had. For a refresher on what counts as a serving, see page 119 in *The Best Life Diet*. And to find out how many servings of grains, fruit, and the other food groups you should have daily (and how many Anything Goes Calories you get), look at the chart on page 119 of the book. (Remember, you can also track your intake and get feedback by joining www.thebestlife.com.)

	Breakfast	Lunch	Dinner	Snack	Other	Other
Grain/Starchy Vegetables						
Fruit						
Vegetables						
Dairy (preferably nonfat or 1%)						
Protein-Rich Foods						
Fat (preferably healthy)						
Anything Goes Calories						

Are your portions becoming more reasonable?   Y   N

NOTES _____

_____

Did you stay within your Anything Goes Calories for treats?   Y   N

NOTES _____

_____

_____

_____

_____

_____

_____

_____

_____

_____

_____

_____

_____

_____

_____

_____

_____

_____

_____

ACTIVITY LEVEL: 0   1   2   3   4   5

Aerobic minutes or steps/day _____

Did you meet your aerobic/step goal?   Y   N

NOTES _____

_____

STRENGTH TRAINING

Exercise								
Weight								
Reps								
Sets								

Did you meet your strength-training goal?   Y   N

NOTES _____

_____

Eating cutoff time: ____ : ____   Bedtime: ____ : ____

Did you cut off eating at least two hours before bedtime?   Y   N

Did you eat three meals (including a nutritious breakfast) and at least one snack?   Y   N

Did you eliminate the six problem foods from your diet?   Y   N

Did you drink at least six 8-ounce glasses of water?   Y   N

Did you take your vitamin supplements?   Y   N

                    TIME

Breakfast   ____ : ____   Hunger rating before eating ____   Hunger rating after eating ____

Lunch   ____ : ____   Hunger rating before eating ____   Hunger rating after eating ____

Dinner   ____ : ____   Hunger rating before eating ____   Hunger rating after eating ____

Snack   ____ : ____   Hunger rating before eating ____   Hunger rating after eating ____

Other meal/snack ____ : ____   Hunger rating before eating ____   Hunger rating after eating ____

Other meal/snack ____ : ____   Hunger rating before eating ____   Hunger rating after eating ____

Did you meet your hunger scale goals?   Y   N

Did you limit your intake of sodium, saturated fat, and added sugar, and eliminate trans fat?   Y   N

NOTES _____

Did you cut back on unhealthy foods and add even more wholesome foods (including whole grains, fruit, vegetables, low-fat dairy, lean protein, and healthy fats) into your diet?   Y   N

NOTES _____

_____

Write down the number of servings you had in each food group. For Anything Goes, just write down the total number of treat calories you had. For a refresher on what counts as a serving, see page 119 in *The Best Life Diet*. And to find out how many servings of grains, fruit, and the other food groups you should have daily (and how many Anything Goes Calories you get), look at the chart on page 119 of the book. (Remember, you can also track your intake and get feedback by joining www.thebestlife.com.)

	Breakfast	Lunch	Dinner	Snack	Other	Other
Grain/Starchy Vegetables						
Fruit						
Vegetables						
Dairy (preferably nonfat or 1%)						
Protein-Rich Foods						
Fat (preferably healthy)						
Anything Goes Calories						

Are your portions becoming more reasonable?   Y   N

NOTES _____

_____

Did you stay within your Anything Goes Calories for treats?   Y   N

NOTES _____

_____

_____

_____

_____

_____

_____

_____

_____

_____

_____

_____

_____

_____

_____

_____

_____

_____

ACTIVITY LEVEL: 0   1   2   3   4   5

Aerobic minutes or steps/day _____

Did you meet your aerobic/step goal?   Y   N

NOTES _____

_____

STRENGTH TRAINING

Exercise							
Weight							
Reps							
Sets							

Did you meet your strength-training goal?   Y   N

NOTES _____

_____

Eating cutoff time: ____:____   Bedtime: ____:____

Did you cut off eating at least two hours before bedtime?   Y   N

Did you eat three meals (including a nutritious breakfast) and at least one snack?   Y   N

Did you eliminate the six problem foods from your diet?   Y   N

Did you drink at least six 8-ounce glasses of water?   Y   N

Did you take your vitamin supplements?   Y   N

                    TIME

Breakfast   ____:____   Hunger rating before eating _____   Hunger rating after eating _____

Lunch   ____:____   Hunger rating before eating _____   Hunger rating after eating _____

Dinner   ____:____   Hunger rating before eating _____   Hunger rating after eating _____

Snack   ____:____   Hunger rating before eating _____   Hunger rating after eating _____

Other meal/snack ____:____   Hunger rating before eating _____   Hunger rating after eating _____

Other meal/snack ____:____   Hunger rating before eating _____   Hunger rating after eating _____

Did you meet your hunger scale goals?   Y   N

Did you limit your intake of sodium, saturated fat, and added sugar, and eliminate trans fat?   Y   N

NOTES _____

_____

Did you cut back on unhealthy foods and add even more wholesome foods (including whole grains, fruit, vegetables, low-fat dairy, lean protein, and healthy fats) into your diet?   Y   N

NOTES _____

_____

Write down the number of servings you had in each food group. For Anything Goes, just write down the total number of treat calories you had. For a refresher on what counts as a serving, see page 119 in *The Best Life Diet*. And to find out how many servings of grains, fruit, and the other food groups you should have daily (and how many Anything Goes Calories you get), look at the chart on page 119 of the book. (Remember, you can also track your intake and get feedback by joining www.thebestlife.com.)

	Breakfast	Lunch	Dinner	Snack	Other	Other
Grain/Starchy Vegetables						
Fruit						
Vegetables						
Dairy (preferably nonfat or 1%)						
Protein-Rich Foods						
Fat (preferably healthy)						
Anything Goes Calories						

Are your portions becoming more reasonable?   Y   N

NOTES _____

_____

Did you stay within your Anything Goes Calories for treats?   Y   N

NOTES _____

_____

_____

_____

_____

_____

_____

_____

_____

_____

_____

_____

_____

_____

_____

_____

ACTIVITY LEVEL: 0   1   2   3   4   5

Aerobic minutes or steps/day _____

Did you meet your aerobic/step goal?   Y   N

NOTES _____

_____

STRENGTH TRAINING

Exercise								
Weight								
Reps								
Sets								

Did you meet your strength-training goal?   Y   N

NOTES _____

_____

Eating cutoff time: ____ : ____   Bedtime: ____ : ____

Did you cut off eating at least two hours before bedtime?   Y   N

Did you eat three meals (including a nutritious breakfast) and at least one snack?   Y   N

Did you eliminate the six problem foods from your diet?   Y   N

Did you drink at least six 8-ounce glasses of water?   Y   N

Did you take your vitamin supplements?   Y   N

                        TIME

Breakfast   ____ : ____   Hunger rating before eating ____   Hunger rating after eating ____

Lunch   ____ : ____   Hunger rating before eating ____   Hunger rating after eating ____

Dinner   ____ : ____   Hunger rating before eating ____   Hunger rating after eating ____

Snack   ____ : ____   Hunger rating before eating ____   Hunger rating after eating ____

Other meal/snack   ____ : ____   Hunger rating before eating ____   Hunger rating after eating ____

Other meal/snack   ____ : ____   Hunger rating before eating ____   Hunger rating after eating ____

Did you meet your hunger scale goals?   Y   N

Did you limit your intake of sodium, saturated fat, and added sugar, and eliminate trans fat?   Y   N

NOTES _____

_____

Did you cut back on unhealthy foods and add even more wholesome foods (including whole grains, fruit, vegetables, low-fat dairy, lean protein, and healthy fats) into your diet?   Y   N

NOTES _____

_____

Write down the number of servings you had in each food group. For Anything Goes, just write down the total number of treat calories you had. For a refresher on what counts as a serving, see page 119 in *The Best Life Diet*. And to find out how many servings of grains, fruit, and the other food groups you should have daily (and how many Anything Goes Calories you get), look at the chart on page 119 of the book. (Remember, you can also track your intake and get feedback by joining www.thebestlife.com.)

	Breakfast	Lunch	Dinner	Snack	Other	Other
Grain/Starchy Vegetables						
Fruit						
Vegetables						
Dairy (preferably nonfat or 1%)						
Protein-Rich Foods						
Fat (preferably healthy)						
Anything Goes Calories						

Are your portions becoming more reasonable?   Y   N

NOTES _____

_____

Did you stay within your Anything Goes Calories for treats?   Y   N

NOTES _____

_____

_____

_____

_____

_____

_____

_____

_____

_____

_____

_____

_____

_____

_____

_____

_____

WEEK: DATE: PHASE 3

ACTIVITY LEVEL: 0   1   2   3   4   5

Aerobic minutes or steps/day _____

Did you meet your aerobic/step goal?   Y   N

NOTES _____

_____

STRENGTH TRAINING

Exercise								
Weight								
Reps								
Sets								

Did you meet your strength-training goal?   Y   N

NOTES _____

Eating cutoff time: _____:_____   Bedtime: _____:_____

Did you cut off eating at least two hours before bedtime?   Y   N

Did you eat three meals (including a nutritious breakfast) and at least one snack?   Y   N

Did you eliminate the six problem foods from your diet?   Y   N

Did you drink at least six 8-ounce glasses of water?   Y   N

Did you take your vitamin supplements?   Y   N

                    TIME
Breakfast   _____:_____   Hunger rating before eating _____ Hunger rating after eating _____

Lunch   _____:_____   Hunger rating before eating _____ Hunger rating after eating _____

Dinner   _____:_____   Hunger rating before eating _____ Hunger rating after eating _____

Snack   _____:_____   Hunger rating before eating _____ Hunger rating after eating _____

Other meal/snack _____:_____   Hunger rating before eating _____ Hunger rating after eating _____

Other meal/snack _____:_____   Hunger rating before eating _____ Hunger rating after eating _____

Did you meet your hunger scale goals?   Y   N

Did you limit your intake of sodium, saturated fat, and added sugar, and eliminate trans fat?   Y   N

NOTES _____

Did you cut back on unhealthy foods and add even more wholesome foods (including whole grains, fruit, vegetables, low-fat dairy, lean protein, and healthy fats) into your diet?   Y   N

NOTES _____

Write down the number of servings you had in each food group. For Anything Goes, just write down the total number of treat calories you had. For a refresher on what counts as a serving, see page 119 in *The Best Life Diet*. And to find out how many servings of grains, fruit, and the other food groups you should have daily (and how many Anything Goes Calories you get), look at the chart on page 119 of the book. (Remember, you can also track your intake and get feedback by joining www.thebestlife.com.)

	Breakfast	Lunch	Dinner	Snack	Other	Other
Grain/Starchy Vegetables						
Fruit						
Vegetables						
Dairy (preferably nonfat or 1%)						
Protein-Rich Foods						
Fat (preferably healthy)						
Anything Goes Calories						

Are your portions becoming more reasonable?　　　　　　　　　　　　　　Y　N

NOTES _____

_____

Did you stay within your Anything Goes Calories for treats?　　　　　　　Y　N

NOTES _____

_____

_____

_____

_____

_____

_____

_____

_____

_____

_____

_____

_____

_____

_____

_____

ACTIVITY LEVEL: 0   1   2   3   4   5

Aerobic minutes or steps/day _____

Did you meet your aerobic/step goal?   Y   N

NOTES _____

_____

STRENGTH TRAINING

Exercise								
Weight								
Reps								
Sets								

Did you meet your strength-training goal?   Y   N

NOTES _____

_____

Eating cutoff time: ____:____   Bedtime: ____:____

Did you cut off eating at least two hours before bedtime?   Y   N

Did you eat three meals (including a nutritious breakfast) and at least one snack?   Y   N

Did you eliminate the six problem foods from your diet?   Y   N

Did you drink at least six 8-ounce glasses of water?   Y   N

Did you take your vitamin supplements?   Y   N

                    TIME

Breakfast   ____:____   Hunger rating before eating ____   Hunger rating after eating ____

Lunch   ____:____   Hunger rating before eating ____   Hunger rating after eating ____

Dinner   ____:____   Hunger rating before eating ____   Hunger rating after eating ____

Snack   ____:____   Hunger rating before eating ____   Hunger rating after eating ____

Other meal/snack   ____:____   Hunger rating before eating ____   Hunger rating after eating ____

Other meal/snack   ____:____   Hunger rating before eating ____   Hunger rating after eating ____

Did you meet your hunger scale goals?   Y   N

Did you limit your intake of sodium, saturated fat, and added sugar, and eliminate trans fat?   Y   N

NOTES _____

_____

Did you cut back on unhealthy foods and add even more wholesome foods (including whole grains, fruit, vegetables, low-fat dairy, lean protein, and healthy fats) into your diet?   Y   N

NOTES _____

_____

Write down the number of servings you had in each food group. For Anything Goes, just write down the total number of treat calories you had. For a refresher on what counts as a serving, see page 119 in *The Best Life Diet*. And to find out how many servings of grains, fruit, and the other food groups you should have daily (and how many Anything Goes Calories you get), look at the chart on page 119 of the book. (Remember, you can also track your intake and get feedback by joining www.thebestlife.com.)

	Breakfast	Lunch	Dinner	Snack	Other	Other
Grain/Starchy Vegetables						
Fruit						
Vegetables						
Dairy (preferably nonfat or 1%)						
Protein-Rich Foods						
Fat (preferably healthy)						
Anything Goes Calories						

Are your portions becoming more reasonable? Y N

NOTES _____

_____

Did you stay within your Anything Goes Calories for treats? Y N

NOTES _____

_____

_____

_____

_____

_____

_____

_____

_____

_____

_____

_____

_____

_____

_____

_____

_____

Weekly Summary

WEEK: _____   PHASE 3

Your weight: _____

Total aerobic minutes/steps for the week _____

Did you meet your aerobic/step goal?   Y N

Did you meet your strength-training goals for the week?   Y N

How many days did you cut off your eating at least two hours before bedtime? _____

How many days did you eat three meals and at least one snack? _____

How many days did you eliminate the six problem foods? _____

How many days did you drink at least six 8-ounce glasses of water? _____

How many days did you take your vitamin supplements? _____

How many days did you meet your hunger scale goals? _____

How many days did you limit your intake of sodium, saturated fat and added
sugar and eliminate trans fat? _____

How many days did you cut back on unhealthy foods and add more wholesome
foods into your diet? _____

How many days did you eat reasonable portions? _____

How many days did you stay within your Anything Goes Calories for treats? _____

How was your week overall? _____

_____

_____

_____

_____

_____

_____

_____

_____

_____

Notes

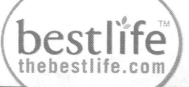